# WHOSE LIFE
## —IS IT—
# ANYHOW?

## DR SIMON L COHEN

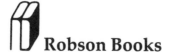
Robson Books

Dedicated to the memory of my mother who
always wanted me to be a doctor.

First published in Great Britain in 1993 by
Robson Books Ltd, Bolsover House, 5-6
Clipstone Street, London W1P 7EB

**British Library Cataloguing in Publication
Data**
A catalogue record for this book is available
from the British Library

ISBN 0 86051 806 X

Photoset in Palatino by Derek Doyle &
Associates, Mold, Clwyd.
Printed in Great Britain by W.B.C. Print and
W.B.C. Bookbinders, Bridgend, Mid-
Glamorgan.

# Contents

*Contents*

# Acknowledgements

I have had invaluable assistance from the staff of Robson Books, who have acted as midwives to this work, especially Louise Dixon.

I would like to thank my sister, Mrs Sheila Brull, who has helped me write this and tried to correct my English. She has shown great patience and perhaps unjustified confidence in my abilities.

Numerous friends and colleagues have advised me. I would especially like to mention Professors Desmond Lawrence and Osmond Reynolds and Doctors N. Wyatt, Mervyn Singer and Rob Miller.

On the spiritual side I have had the benefit of advice from my first teacher and the pioneer of modern interest in Jewish Medical Ethics, Chief Rabbi Lord Jakobovits. The Reverend Professor Boyd also allowed me time to discuss Christian Medical Ethics, as did the various chaplains of University College Hospital. Professor C. Miriam Campanini has read the manuscript and made many helpful suggestions both regarding legal aspects and the general content of the book, which have been invaluable.

This would not have been possible without all the kind help and patience of my secretary, Mrs Berti Rooke-Ley. Finally, thanks to my wife, Yael, for her constant support and reminders to me to finish the work.

# Foreword

This book is written in an attempt to inform the public of the ethical dilemmas encountered in intensive care treatment and to elicit public support to ensure continuing adequate intensive care life saving facilities.

It is written at a time of great uncertainty about the future of medical care, particularly in the inner cities. Hospitals and units are being amalgamated, rationalized and closed. Morale is low. Financial pressures are a prime cause for changes in the delivery of health care, and facilities for intensive care may be threatened.

The Tomlinson Report on the provision of health care in inner London suggested wholesale closures and the reorganization of London teaching hospitals, with more resources going to the improvement of primary and community care. My fear is that the money will be saved by enacting the closures with attendant redundancy of staff and deteriorating service for the public. I also suspect that the money to improve primary and community care in London will either not be provided at all or granted in a slow and haphazard manner.

There has been a great increase in public concern about medical ethical issues in Britain in recent years, and the trend is for these problems to be resolved by the courts, as has happened for many years in the United States. One celebrated action in 1992 concerned the tragic case of Tony Bland, in a persistent vegetative state for over three years following injury at the Hillsborough football disaster in 1989. All concerned parties – the health authority, Mr

Bland's parents and his doctor – wanted to withdraw nasogastric feeding from. However the local coroner warned that the doctor could face prosecution for murder if he discontinued feeding or antibiotics. The case came to the High Court's Family Division, who declared that artificial nutrition and hydration and any other medical support measures may be withdrawn. This case ably highlights the ethical, moral and legal problems faced by the doctor who can withdraw treatment but then may have to face consequences such as accusations of negligence or even murder. It is hoped that higher court decisions will clarify the position. It is a major concern that every similar tragic case – and there are many – may have to be adjudicated in court with the attendant anguish for all concerned.

I trained as a General Hospital Physician with a special interest in kidney disease. Through my work with patients undergoing kidney transplants I developed an interest in the problems of people facing acute medical crisis. This book has inevitably been influenced by my own personal background and experience – and, no doubt, by my private convictions and prejudices. In an attempt to counter this, I have canvassed the views of many of my colleagues, and the case histories that illustrate the problems of intensive care have been taken from a number of units in addition to my own. I try to present a balanced view of the achievements and failings of intensive care, along with its needs and contributions.

The relationship between doctor and patient is changing, and the days of the omnipotent doctor, able to make decisions of life and death without consulting the patient or his family, are all but over. It is against this background that this book is written. My hope is that it will go some way towards informing the public of the many and various issues, and allow them to make their own decisions in these dilemmas – literally of life and death – in the intensive care unit.

# Introduction

The intensive care unit (ICU) is the place in a hospital where the most critically ill patients are treated. It is a stage on which many dramas of life and death are enacted. The aim of this book is to acquaint the general reader with some of the problems of intensive care and with some of the formidably difficult ethical problems the work presents not only to the medical profession but also to the public.

In the past few years the fierce political arguments about the nature, organization and funding of Britain's National Health Service have, if nothing else, left no one in any doubt about the truly enormous cost of maintaining even the most basic levels of care. Intensive care, which involves some of the most concentrated, specialized and 'high-tech' work in a hospital, is hugely expensive even by the standards of the service. Some of the ethical challenges that confront the staff of an intensive care unit almost daily are bound up with the problems of finance.

These challenges intensify year by year because of the ever-increasing sophistication and cost of medical technology, combined with an ageing population which demands that the most advanced methods of treatment be available to all. This simply cannot be reconciled with the finite resources governments are prepared to devote to the public health service. Hospitals are required to run on very tight budgets, which can and does lead to the trimming of services. Hospital management may face the the stark choice of spending £100,000 to keep a hopelessly damaged individual in intensive care for two months, or allowing him to die and possibly spending the money on four kidney transplants.

Other ethical problems, equally intractable, have to do with the ways in which respect for the sanctity of life may lead an intensive care team to prolong unduly the inexorable process of dying of a patient who is terminally ill. They may give a new and bitter twist to the couplet in Arthur Hugh Clough's reworking of the Decalogue:

Thou shalt not kill; but need'st not strive
Officiously to keep alive.

It is possible, with life-support machines, to keep severely brain-damaged people in what is called a 'persistent vegetative state' for a long time. Whether it is desirable to do so is another matter; and, once started, when should such life support be withdrawn – and who should be responsible for taking the decision to withdraw it? The fears and anxieties occasioned by the technically remarkable feats of intensive care underlay the passing of the Patient Self Determination Act in the United States. This act requires hospitals to inform patients, on admission, that they may prepare a 'living will' specifying their preferences for terminal care, including life support, and proxy arrangements for making decisions.

It is recognized that Great Britain is underprovided in intensive care services compared with other advanced Western countries. I know from bitter experience that trying to find places for patients in intensive care and struggling to make the best use of limited resources is a daily task. Who to treat: who to deny treatment to? 'First come, first served'? But that might result in filling the ICU with terminally ill patients, so denying the chance of recovery to others who are gravely ill but who need more limited support. The public benefits from the work of our intensive care units. So it should: it pays for them, after all.

# 1

# The Intensive Care Unit at Work

In 1989 the King's Fund, an independent British organization whose work includes the study of health-care policy, produced a report on intensive care in the United Kingdom. The report defined intensive care as a service for patients with potentially curable diseases who can benefit from more detailed observation and treatment than is normally available in the general wards and departments of a hospital. It has been only during the past 30 years or so that intensive care units (ICUs) have become an established part of hospitals throughout the National Health Service. And such are the constraints on resources and staff in NHS hospitals that in practice only the most critically ill patients qualify for intensive care in Britain.

'Critically ill' in such cases means that at least one of the body's organ systems has broken down, and ICUs owe their origin largely to the development of emergency treatments for such failed systems. The coronary care units in hospitals, for instance, specialize in the emergency measures developed by medical teams for dealing with heart attacks and cardiac arrest, when a patient's heart stops even though he or she might have no record of heart disease. Another milestone in the development of intensive care was the poliomyelitis epidemic of the 1950s. One of the effects of a severe attack was to paralyse the muscles that control breathing, and the invention of the mechanical ventilator saved the lives of many polio victims.

As these and other treatments and technology were developed and became widely available, it seemed logical to concentrate the most critically ill patients in a separate part of a hospital, where specialists and highly trained nurses could devote all their time to them. And so the first ICUs appeared. Over the years many units have tended to specialize in various ways – some, for instance, in the treatment of specific organ systems (heart, kidneys, liver or whatever), others in specific types of treatment, such as chemotherapy for cancer, or in particular categories of patient (newborn babies, for instance, or children). The larger hospitals may have a number of such specialized units. On the other hand, reasons of funding and resources have meant that in many hospitals patients suffering from a variety of serious illnesses or injuries may all be treated in a 'mixed' ICU. This is the case with my own hospital in central London.

The work of any two mixed ICUs may differ widely because each unit necessarily reflects the activities of the hospital in which it is located – and hospitals differ in the special services they offer. Geographical location influences the type of work undertaken by many hospitals; those in areas of heavy industry or motorways, for instance, tend to get the most accident cases. Again, an ICU in a hospital which has a major cardiac surgery unit will obviously devote much of its time to treating patients with serious heart problems.

### Who gets intensive care?

No hard and fast rules govern selection of patients for intensive care. And the decision not to select a certain patient is not by any means always made on strictly medical grounds. In the NHS, constraints such as lack of equipment and shortage of trained nurses or other staff play a significant part, as we shall see later. And then, of course, a patient has to be referred by his or her consultant – and the attitude of the consultant in charge may determine whether or not a patient is transferred to intensive care. A consultant may come to the conclusion that the ICU has not much to offer a particular patient. I have even come across consultants who genuinely believe that sending a patient to intensive care would amount to an admission of failure on their part. On the other hand, I have known staff of ICUs to openly criticize primary physicians or surgeons for supposedly faulty diagnosis or treatment of serious illness – and that is hardly likely to encourage a spirit of cooperation between the various medical teams. I once worked in a hospital where the only patients sent to intensive care were those whom the admitting consultant was certain were going to die – as if the sole purpose of the highly trained team of specialists and support staff and all their vastly expensive equipment was to ease the passage of patients into the grave.

Since intensive care is enormously expensive, and since the number and resources of ICUs are finite, one occasionally hears the argument that those who, in one way or another, are responsible for their own illnesses or injuries should enjoy a lower priority for treatment than other patients. Alcoholics, who are susceptible to potentially lethal head injuries, drug addicts, who often develop metabolic complications of muscle break-down due to lying unconscious and immobile for long periods, and those indulging in solvent abuse are typical examples.

Intensive care can tackle such problems – though not the addictions themselves, nor the social and psychological problems that cause them. AIDS sufferers are among the latest patients to fall into this group, and it is predicted that they will arrive in intensive care in ever-growing numbers in the next few years. It is essential that the staff of ICUs are totally unprejudiced in their attitudes to patients whose problems are supposedly self-inflicted. Neither perceived social inadequacy nor even criminality is morally acceptable grounds for denying a patient intensive care.

## Life and death decisions

The decision of when to stop resuscitation of a patient who is clearly going to die if he is denied further intensive care lies at the heart of one of the ethical dilemmas facing the staff of an ICU. There are occasions when any further attempts to restart a patient's heart would be nothing less than pointless assaults on his dignity. This is often the case with patients who have terminal cancer. Equally, however, for many people there is something objectionable in the idea of the doctor in charge playing God and handing down decisions as to who will and who will not be resuscitated. There have been notorious cases of 'DNR' ('Do not resuscitate') notices being attached to the clipboard notes at the end of the beds of elderly patients.

The doctor's role in making a decision about if and when to stop support must be purely a medical one: to determine whether or not resuscitation can succeed and, if it can, what sort of quality of life will be possible for the patient. And even then the decision whether and when to switch off the support systems must, where possible, be made in consultation with the patient's dependants or proxies.

The trouble is that it is often very difficult to be certain that a patient will survive or will die under particular circumstances. Just how difficult – and therefore how tricky the ethical problem can be – is demonstrated by a recent case in the ICU at my own hospital. It concerned a 67-year-old man who had experienced severe depression since his wife had died three years before. During this time he suffered acute back pains. He had consulted a number of specialists, and eventually convinced a neurosurgeon that he should have an operation.

This passed off uneventfully; but on the tenth day in the neurosurgical unit he began to suffer extreme pain in the abdomen. As this unit was not geared to treat him for this, he was transferred to our ICU, where he received intensive care while a long debate ensued as to the nature and cause of this complication. It soon emerged that he had septicaemia (acute blood poisoning), which was causing a major upset to his blood pressure and most of his bodily systems. But what was causing the septicaemia?

He had a history of diverticular disease of the large intestine. And it was suggested that the acute abdominal symptoms might have been due to disease of the lungs – respiratory conditions may cause pain to be transferred to the abdomen. A second operation revealed nothing abnormal apart from a distended gall bladder; but shortly afterwards his wound burst and he required a third operation.

He now developed profound weakness of the limbs – a common enough symptom in patients who undergo prolonged intensive care. He was, in fact, in the ICU for over six weeks, and throughout this period was fed intravenously. Not surprisingly, he remained very confused mentally and his underlying depression persisted.

Eventually, after his physical condition showed no sign of improvement, his sisters (who were his nearest relatives) requested that treatment be discontinued. But then, after repeated examinations and tests, it was found that he had some gallstones in the common bile duct. These were removed by a method that does not require surgery – and the patient eventually made a good recovery.

Why did we persist in treating this patient who, over a

long period of intensive care, showed no sign of recovery and whose next of kin had resigned themselves to his death? We had long discussions and arguments over the case. Obviously, part of the explanation is that the staff of an ICU hate to lose a patient, especially to a complaint or series of complaints that they cannot even identify. Our persistence in this case, however, arose mainly from the fact that the patient showed no evidence of malignant disease (this type of gall bladder disease, which nowadays is readily treatable, occurs mainly in very sick patients and is very difficult to diagnose). But the whole episode demonstrates how it is quite possible to give up on patients who in fact have the capacity to make a full recovery.

Most patients in an ICU require intensive care for 24 hours or less, but much can be achieved in such a relatively short time. For instance, both the kidneys and the lungs may be severely damaged on an acute short-term basis and yet recover fully if they receive prompt intensive care. And although complete recovery in such cases may take weeks or months, the most critical phase of the recovery process will have been the few hours the patient spent in intensive care.

There is a clear distinction between this example and that of a patient who, it becomes clear, cannot possibily survive in spite of all the support the ICU can bring to bear on his behalf. In such a case, we do not switch off the life-support machines, but the treatment is scaled down, the patient's comfort is assured, and the next of kin counselled. Any further complications in his condition, such as new infections or falling blood pressure, are not specifically treated, and the patient is allowed gradually to fade away.

It could be argued that this is nothing more nor less than passive euthanasia; and certainly if it were spelt out as policy it would be ethically questionable, to say the least. After all, how can we be sure that a patient might not survive if we strove harder and more effectively? A patient whose chance of recovery seems hopeless today might be effectively treated by new techniques that become available in the months ahead.

### Technology and the dignity of the patient

Intensive care nowadays relies heavily on a formidable array of high-technology machinery. Some, such as the mechanical ventilator to aid breathing and the balloon pump to augment the heart beat, act as stand-ins for bodily organs or muscle systems that are temporarily out of action. Others, which monitor all the operations of the patient's organ systems, help both in diagnosis of disease and measurement of the progress of recovery. The latest machines computerize all the measurements of bodily functions and produce graphic displays on monitor screens by the patient's bedside.

In this area, too, ethical questions intrude. There is a growing danger in the most technologically sophisticated ICUs that the patient may seem to be merely the subject of physiological experiments and that it is forgotten that at the other end of that tangle of wires and tubes is a human being whose very survival is balanced on a knife edge. Often a patient may be unable to communicate with doctors and nurses or with his relatives because he has tubes in his mouth or is heavily sedated. It might be argued that patients under sedation are unaware of any loss of dignity; but members of a patient's family and other visiting relatives are often distressed by the sight of their unconscious loved one attached to a frightening array of hardware.

Sedation, incidentally, gives rise to another problem. Most patients undergoing intensive care are heavily sedated in order to ease the pain or extreme discomfort occasioned by the treatment they are undergoing. It is difficult for the ICU to determine whether or not the

patient is in distress, but careful sedation with tran-
quillizers may be important in the recovery phase from
full life-support in intensive care. The problem is that too
much sedation may delay recovery and so prolong
dependence on machines such as the mechanical
ventilator. So a balance must be struck between the
comfort and dignity of the patient and the need to obtain,
often by invasive monitoring, accurate information about
bodily functions.

Finally, there is the occasional suspicion, however
unjustified, that prolonged attempts by the staff of an ICU
to overcome impossible odds, such as terminal cancer, are
inspired as much by the interests of medical research as by
the welfare of the patient. And the uncomfortable fact that
significant advances in medical knowledge have indeed
resulted from heroic but obviously foredoomed attempts
of this kind do nothing to allay such suspicion.

All human life is of equal and infinite value, and the
staff of an ICU must approach their work from this ethical
position. Unfortunately, health-care resources are finite,
intensive care is extremely expensive, and ICUs are
limited in size and number. The question arises as to
whether one can justify, as a basic principle of policy,
spending a very large proportion of one's public health
resources on a very small number of patients. And if one
can, who is to determine priorities? Who is to define the
criteria for admission to intensive care? Are the doctors to
be trusted? Who is qualified to pronounce whether or not
intensive care is in a patient's interests if he himself is
unable to communicate? Can it ever be in the patient's
interests to die? These are profoundly difficult questions,
but it is important that we, as members of the general
public, as well as the medical profession and the health
authorities, address them seriously and with open minds.

# 2

# The Organization of an ICU

Intensive care units provide a quality and concentration of care for patients that is not possible in other departments of a hospital. There is a much higher staff to patient ratio in the ICU than elsewhere. Ideally there should be a fully qualified intensive care nurse at the bedside of each patient in the unit all the time. Because of the shift structure of the nursing day, each patient would require three nurses for any given 24-hour period.

Intensive care nurses are highly skilled; they will have had several years of postgraduate training, and most will have undertaken special courses in intensive care. In the unit they are supported by more junior nurses, who carry out the less specialized tasks.

A doctor should be present in the ICU throughout the 24 hours, working a shift system similar to the nurses'. Unfortunately, this level of manning is not always achieved, and it is a matter of concern that a doctor may be on duty overnight, with little rest and no sleep, and then be required to undertake exceptionally difficult and quite possibly life-saving procedures on patients the following day.

In recent years there has been a shift in the relative status of doctors and nurses in the ICU. The nurse is no longer regarded as the handmaiden of the doctor but as an independent, highly qualified professional. The changing relationship between the two has led on occasion to argument as to who is actually in charge of the unit. The important thing, of course, is that doctors, nurses and the rest of the staff should work as a team.

## Layout of the unit

Intensive care units vary considerably in size, depending on the size of the hospitals in which they are located. There are obvious economic advantages in having one very large central ICU rather than several smaller ones in a given area. The strictly medical advantages of such an arrangement are more open to doubt. In any case, the hospital service has not developed in this way in the United Kingdom, where there are commonly quite a number of small hospitals rather than a few big ones in the major cities. Often, each of these smaller hospitals will have its own ICU. If these were closed in favour of one or two much larger ones, there would be a constant problem of having to move critically ill patients from the smaller hospitals to one of the central ICUs.

Whether it is capable of handling few or many patients, it is vital that an ICU has plenty of room. Each of the beds in the unit needs to have much more space around it than a bed in one of the general wards. Ease of access is important because a variety of machines may need to be brought quickly to the bedside – ventilators, dialysis or other emergency equipment, X-ray, ultrasound and other imaging machines, and monitoring devices to take constant measurements of the patient's vital functions. A range of services, including piped oxygen, suction equipment, and automated pumps used to deliver accurate intravenous doses of essential drugs should be available at the head of each bed.

One quarter to one third of the beds in the unit should

be in cubicles to avoid the possibility of infections passing from one patient to another. Patients whose immune system is malfunctioning, or those without white cells in the blood, must be isolated to reduce the chance of their being infected by harmful bacteria. Patients in intensive care sometimes develop infection with organisms resistant to the usual run of antibiotics. For instance, repeated treatment with antibiotics may allow the selecting out of unusually resistant bacteria, and patients carrying such organisms are potentially a hazard to others undergoing intensive care. In such cases, it is the patients carrying the resistant organisms who are isolated in cubicles.

In the United States, an ICU typically has about 5 per cent of the total number of beds in a hospital. In Europe the figure is more like 1 or 2 per cent. A survey by Professor J.L. Vincent of attitudes towards ethical problems in intensive care medicine showed that a shortage of beds is common in Europe, and particularly in the United Kingdom.*

In view of this, it is ironic that it may happen that an ICU is declared full even though some of its beds are empty. The usual reason for this is that there are not enough nurses or other personnel to staff the beds. The question then arises of what to do with a new arrival who needs intensive care. He can either be put on a ventilator and 'parked' in a corridor until another patient is fit enough to be moved out of the ICU; or he can be sent on a potentially hazardous journey to a unit in another hospital.

Shortage of highly trained nurses can have damaging consequences for the unit. In the short term, insufficient nurses will inevitably result in those on the staff overworking at times when the unit is at its busiest. This can lead to inefficiency and perhaps dangerous errors; and this, in turn, will cause job dissatisfaction and may

---

* Vincent, J.L., 'European attitudes to ethics in ICU medicine', *Intensive Care Medicine* (1990), 16 (4), 256–64.

result in resignations – which of course will simply make the problem worse.

## Integrating intensive care operations

There is no simple answer to the 'house full' dilemma in the ICU. In a large hospital a quite common solution is to transfer the fittest patient in the ICU to another of the hospital's specialized departments: the high dependency unit. This unit provides a higher category of care than is possible in the general wards, but its staff-to-patient ratio (about 1:2) is not as high as that in an ICU. In the normal course of events many patients graduate from the ICU to a high dependency unit, so it is usual for the two units to be sited close together within the hospital building. One of the criteria that determine the move from intensive care to high dependency is that the patient has less need of life-support equipment and other machines.

The recovery unit is the third and least invasive of the three centres of activity that, ideally, should be fully integrated within the operation of intensive care. Here patients are taken after undergoing surgery. It is possible to ventilate patients in the recovery unit, but often only on a short-term basis as the units are open only from 9 am to 5 pm. Astonishing as it may seem, many hospitals in the NHS do not have recovery units. The patients in recovery are at a lower level of dependency than those in the ICU or high dependency unit, but the staff here are equipped to maintain the patient's airway and to monitor blood pressure and circulation, and the unit plays a vital role in averting post-operative disasters.

In an ideal world there would, obviously, be ready access to the ICU from casualty or emergency department and from the operating theatres – but this is not always achieved. If a critically ill patient has to be moved to an ICU in another hospital, it is essential that his condition is stabilized first; and he should be accompanied by an ICU doctor trained and fully competent in resuscitation techniques.

## The self-sufficient unit

A well-designed ICU does not skimp on space in its non-clinical areas. Education and study are rightly regarded by staff members as essential ongoing activities, and the unit should have good-sized rooms for seminars which the staff of other departments in the hospital should also be encouraged to attend. Other basic requirements are comfortable rest rooms for the staff, a doctor's bedroom, rooms in which patients' relatives can be interviewed and counselled, and ample storage facilities for drugs and equipment and for notes and records.

Accurate note-taking and record-keeping are central to the operation of the unit because they allow critical analysis of the effects of every stage in the complex interventionary procedures involved in intensive care. This is important not only for efficient clinical management and research; it also furnishes reliable evidence if there is an unfortunate mishap or medical accident to a patient undergoing intensive care. Both the doctors and the nurses make their own separate reports, although there is a case for a unified, perhaps computerized single record. At present the nurse's record is more complete than the doctor's notes. The 1989 King's Fund report (see p.25) recommended that each ICU codify its clinical policy in the form of written guidelines. In the unit where I work we have developed a book of clinical algorithms, or procedure guidelines, for just this purpose. But it is obvious that it would be enormously helpful if intensivists throughout the National Health Service could agree on which data (clinical and economic) should be collected and in what form. This would not only help individual units to compare their experiences with those of others; it would also make it easier for researchers to compare and evaluate specific practices of different units, especially in areas where expert opinions differ about the best methods and procedures.

It is also important that ICUs share their expertise and findings with personnel in other departments of the hospital. This can lead to improvements in clinical procedures in the general wards. One example of this is the latest approach to heart failure. Until quite recently the first treatment has always been administering a diuretic, which increases urine flow, to relieve congestion of the lungs. It is largely through studies of patients in intensive care that specialists have come to realize that in many cases the problem is not one of congestion or overload but of the maldistribution of fluid within the body. It follows that drugs designed to redistribute blood may be more effective in these cases than diuretics.

It has been suggested that, in view of the shortage of the most highly trained nurses in many units, the numbers and skill mix of nurses and the particular tasks each carries out on every case should be recorded. Sometimes the division of work between the ICU and related units may not make for the best, or at least the most economical, use of nursing resources. For instance, a patient in a high dependency unit who has just come off the ventilator in intensive care may be able to breathe spontaneously, but he is likely to be restless and agitated. He will now require a good deal more nursing time and attention than if he had been able to remain sedated and on the ventilator in the ICU for a little while longer. Any commonsense measures that help to alleviate the pressure on frequently overworked staff are welcome, but cost-effectiveness and convenience cannot be allowed to override the best interests of the patient.

# 3

# Clinical Challenges

Only desperately ill patients come to the intensive care unit – a situation that offers a tremendous challenge and sometimes inspiration to the doctors and nurses working in the unit. Sometimes we fail; sometimes we can be criticized for continuing treatment too long; but the chance to restore a mortally sick person to a full and active life is a great spur. It carries with it tremendous responsibility, and sometimes we over-estimate our ability to enable a patient to survive.

Although intensive care is about the artificial support of failing body systems, often with the aid of sophisticated machines, the greatest challenge for the doctor may be to exercise diagnostic skill. This is especially the case, for instance, if a patient, while exhibiting no obvious symptoms, is clearly not progressing as well as expected. The experienced intensive care doctor may diagnose infection correctly on these grounds. An example was that of a woman of 55, on holiday from Scandinavia, who suffered an acute abdominal catastrophe: she perforated a stomach ulcer. An immediate operation was carried out as an emergency, and her abdominal cavity was found to be soiled by the contents of her stomach. After the operation she required treatment in intensive care, with the usual paraphernalia of fluid replacement and ventilation. Her condition simply did not seem to stabilize. It is routine that patients treated with artificial ventilation have a stomach tube in place to make sure that the stomach is kept empty and there is no possibility of aspiration of its contents into the lungs. In this case, the stomach aspirations were of large volume. Tests also showed that her blood contained an excessive proportion of acid – an ominous sign – in spite of having the proper replacement of fluids and ventilation. The experienced intensivist who saw her immediately summoned the surgeons because he felt that the only rational explanation for the situation was continuing leakage from the stomach. This proved to be the case; a second operation was done immediately, and the patient made a good recovery. Had these signs not been so promptly recognized the patient's condition might have continued to deteriorate, with the development of multiple organ system failure and death. Unexplained excess acid levels developing in a patient in intensive care frequently indicates infection.

Similarly if a patient is infected and the source is unknown the explanation may be that there has been an acute abdominal catastrophe, often without any of the classical clinical signs. We have had to pressurize surgeons to operate on these patients.

A further example occurred in a man who sustained a fractured pelvis following a fall from the fourth floor. His progress was slow, with abnormally low blood pressure and a brownish discharge from one of the wound sites where pins had been inserted to stabilize his pelvis. Finally, after three and a half weeks, the wounds and the abdomen were explored, revealing a tear of the colon (large bowel) with an associated abscess. He rapidly improved following the operation.

A major problem for the recipients of kidney transplants is that they have to be treated continuously with cortisone-like drugs and others similar to those used in chemotherapy, whose side effects include depression of the immune system. As a result of this, organisms which are the normal inhabitants of the body surfaces become opportunistic pathogens, causing severe infections.

A girl, aged 22, had received a kidney transplant from her mother four years prior to her final illness. She became ill for three months in her home in a Third World country, where no definitive diagnosis was reached. She came to London in a desperate condition and eventually we were able to demonstrate that she had nocardiosis, a very rare bacterial infection that occurs only in people whose immune defences are seriously impaired.

She was treated for nine days in the intensive care unit, during all of which time she was unconscious. We knew that she had nocardia meningitis (inflammation of the membranes surrounding the brain) and that the known results of treating this condition are appalling, as it has a very high mortality rate. However, we worked in close conjunction with our microbiologists who, having made this diagnosis, encouraged our hopes that by the application of the most appropriate antibiotics we could pull her through, in spite of the evidence that she was deteriorating every day. She required mechanical ventilation throughout this period. She had no white cells in her blood and she gradually lost all signs of evidence of activity of her brain. We went through a formalistic set of tests to see if her brain was dead, and at that moment she stopped all forms of life activity. This was a horrifying experience for the team involved in the test. Perhaps we should have trusted our own judgement of the inevitable course of events. However, the challenge to try to save the life of a young girl is something that we could not easily refuse. Sometimes, as described in a later case, profoundly ill patients do recover from meningitis.

## The challenge of leukaemia

In our institution we see numbers of patients with acute leukaemia. This often occurs in young patients. The treatment possibilities in these patients have greatly expanded in recent years and results of bone marrow transplants have become extremely good. It is, as with other situations, only the rare patient who actually requires the support of intensive care. Put another way, our success rate is 90 per cent for bone marrow transplants; our intensive care unit tries to increase that rate to 92 per cent. Sometimes the challenge provided by this effort may be thought to be inappropriate or too prolonged. But the stakes are very high.

The treatment basically consists of, first, destroying the bone marrow where, in leukaemia, there is a malignant over-production of white blood cells and, second, restoring the bone marrow later by a transplant to produce normal white cells.

A 13-year-old boy was diagnosed as having acute myelomonocytic leukaemia, a particularly vicious form of the disease known to have a very bad prognosis. The haematologists felt that the patient would either die or recover within the first week. He came to us with failure of both lungs and kidneys and with evidence of widespread internal bleeding. He was treated with ventilation and haemofiltration, and was kept alive for some 16 days in this way.

In cases like this there is no question that the family would want us to persist over and above any time that we felt logically the patient might experience benefit. He developed increasing evidence of pneumonia, and his blood pressure faded away in spite of support. His unfortunate parents maintained a vigil throughout the illness. When he died, his parents asked that he be dressed in his school uniform, perhaps reflecting their Chinese cultural customs.

When patients undergo bone marrow transplants, it is part of the procedure that their own bone marrow is first ablated with irradiation. Unfortunately, if the bone marrow transplant does not 'take', the white cell count will remain low, with the inevitable consequence that the patient is a prey to infection. It is especially dangerous if patients have respiratory problems when they have no white cells. We have seen cases where chemotherapy, which is given as part of the work-up for bone marrow transplantation, affects the function of the heart. Theoretically it is possible that the bone marrow, heart, lungs and kidneys may all recover after failing, but usually such combined failure proves fatal. The hope is that the marrow will recover and, engrafted with the reappearance of white cells, will enable the patient to fight the infection.

Another clinical challenge with increasing ethical overtones was provided by an unfortunate 29-year-old woman who first developed acute lymphatic leukaemia at the age of 22. She was treated with standard chemotherapy and her condition stabilized. This remission lasted for five years. She was then treated again with chemotherapy and remitted once more and at this stage received a bone marrow transplant from a fully matched sibling donor. This was complicated by acute and then chronic graft versus host disease (GVH). This is a condition where the donor blood cells mount an immunological attack against the host, which is manifested by skin, liver and gut problems.

She was able to go home but was admitted to hospital locally with septicaemia from a pneumonia. This responded to antibiotics, but a few days after discharge she rapidly became unwell and collapsed. She came into hospital with a very high fever, in a state of shock with low blood pressure.

During the next 24 hours she developed rapidly progressive kidney and respiratory failure, culminating in a cardiac arrest. She was resuscitated from this and treated with ventilation and haemofiltration. At that time she developed an extensive rash all over her arms and legs. This was thought to be due to recurrent septicaemia. Unfortunately it now became clear that, owing to a combination of small blood vessel blockage and low blood pressure, her legs were not viable, and were becoming gangrenous owing to the damaged blood supply. During this time she had evidence of malfunction of the heart as well.

The gangrenous legs were contributing to her desperate toxic state. The vascular surgeons concluded that there was no prospect for recovery of the blood supply to the legs and that her life depended on their amputation. Fortunately she made a good recovery from the operation, and her general condition greatly improved. She was able to regain her cardiac, respiratory and renal function over the course of the next two to three weeks, and later was discharged home.

This case was remarkable in that she was able to recover in spite of having at least four organ systems failing – heart, lungs and kidneys as well as her underlying disorder, which in fact was thought to be in remission at the time – in addition to the terrible catastrophe of the gangrenous legs.

The decision to carry out amputations was not an easy one because of the disability it would leave her, and at the time it seemed that her prospects of survival were not great. However, we did not feel that we would add to her suffering by removing the legs and considered (correctly, as it turned out) that the operation might well result in considerable benefit. Her family and the patient supported us in this decision and gave consent to the operation. Probably the key factor which allowed this patient to survive as against many others in similar situations, perhaps with seemingly less severe initial problems, who did not, was that her bone marrow transplant was functioning and these white cells were able to give her some ability to respond to treatment and to protect her from infection. It is this kind of case which encourages us to try so hard with leukaemic patients. Prolonging the life of a 29-year-old, even at the price of disability, must be worthwhile. She was able to return home, but she died there three months later, unfortunately, of another infection.

## Heart disease

In recent times there have been some exciting developments in drug treatment of heart disease. A drug called captopril has been shown to be of benefit in patients severely limited in their activity by heart failure. Unfortunately under certain conditions this family of drugs, called ACE (angiotensin-converting enzyme) inhibitors, can cause kidney damage and even failure.

A 67-year-old lady with a history of heart disease had only one kidney, her other one having been removed some years previously after it developed a tumour. When she was given the ACE inhibitor her heart failure greatly improved but she developed failure of her one remaining kidney. She required treatment in intensive care to adjust her fluid balance and stabilize the combined cardiac and renal problems.

After some days of juggling with her medication it was decided to investigate more deeply the causes of her renal failure. A radioisotopic technique to measure kidney function suggested that the blood flow into the single kidney was restricted. This was confirmed by angiography X-ray of the artery, which showed that the entrance of the artery was narrowed. The radiologist decided, after consultation with us, to expand this narrowing which was the cause of her intolerance to the ACE inhbitor. The technique, called angioplasty, was carried out with great success.

The decision to attempt angioplasty was difficult. If the angioplasty had not gone well she might have lost what little function she had in that single kidney and required chronic dialysis, but it is very doubtful if she would have been accepted by a dialysis programme in the United Kingdom because of her cardiac state and age. Dialysis facilities in Britain are still limited compared to those in other Western countries. Fortunately, the angioplasty resulted in the improvement of her kidney function and in her ability to tolerate the ACE inhibitor.

As a result of these aggressive investigations and the proper application of intensive care this woman now leads an active life helped by an ACE inhibitor which she continues to tolerate well.

Another technique of cardiac intensive care that may be life saving is insertion of a pacemaker to speed the ineffectively functioning, pathologically slow heart. Alterations in heart rhythm are potentially fatal but are eminently curable by proper treatment. New drugs are being introduced to support the flagging, failing heart, and the physical balloon pump system is also widely used. Acute surgery, including even heart transplantation, has a vital place, but facilities for this are limited in the United Kingdom.

The art of medicine is at least in part the ability to recognize unusual patterns of symptoms or signs and to try to treat them. This may be literally a matter of life and death in the intensive care unit. A recent example occurred when a patient who was progressing well deteriorated over a few hours: he became short of breath, stopped passing urine and his blood pressure fell in spite of his receiving intravenous fluid. Fortunately we realized that fluid was accumulating in the sac around the heart, impairing the heart's action. We were able to remove this fluid and he went on to recover. The ability to recognize and treat this sort of acute medical emergency represents another clinical challenge: the doctor in intensive care needs to be first and foremost a good clinician.

Another patient who provided us with a great challenge – and finally great satisfaction – was a 19-year-old American student who suddenly became ill and developed uncontrollable epilepsy. It was felt that this was caused by viral encephalitis, a virus infection of the brain. The prognosis in encephalitis is often very poor, although the diagnosis is difficult to substantiate.

The problem was that the fits continued and continued. She required full ventilation because the massive amounts of drugs given to control the epilepsy interfered with her ability to breathe. In fact it was only by paralysing her and ventilating her that control was at all possible. This perilous situation continued for around six weeks, with her parents maintaining a vigil at the bedside.

During this time a variety of complications occurred. She developed pancreatitis (inflammation of the pancreas), a side effect of one of the drugs which were essential to keep her alive. This in turn was life threatening, as was a bout of septicaemia complicated by renal failure, probably related to the intravenous lines that she needed. The challenge was whether or not to continue our efforts. We did not know if she would recover and if she did would she be brain-damaged. It was her youth and the lack of unequivocal evidence that recovery was impossible which encouraged us to continue. Eventually she slowly recovered. After three months in intensive care she was able to return home to her studies!

### Multiple organ system failure

A challenge of a different type is that required to deal with multiple organ system failure (MOSF), which occurs as a result of many overwhelming illnesses. The final pattern of organ failures is often the same regardless of whether it was initiated by infections, burns or trauma. This suggests the pathways of organ failure may be common, or that the same type of biochemical substances (mediators) occur in all these conditions. One of the greatest problems of intensive care is to prevent organ failure. There is a great deal of work in progress to study these mediators and to attempt to counteract them in various ways, for instance by developing antibodies to the mediators or by blocking their actions with antibodies to their receptors. This would seem a better approach than the present one of empirically supporting the failed organs. Unfortunately, we do not know which mediators and receptors are the most significant. Often the trigger for MOSF is infection. Early recognition and prompt treatment of infection is critical in saving life. It would be enormously helpful if we could discover methods of enhancing the ability of white blood cells to fight against infection.

Hopefully just as the development of effective drug treatment for tuberculosis eliminated the need for sanatoriums, so better understanding of organ failure mechanisms may reduce the need for intensive care.

# 4

# Who Qualifies for Intensive Care?

It is a matter of debate as to which patients should be treated in intensive care and how much benefit they should receive. In an attempt to answer these questions the King's Fund convened a multidisciplinary panel. They reported on 'Intensive Care in the United Kingdom' and suggested criteria for admission to the ICU. They stated that, primarily, intensive care should be given in the expectation of beneficial consequences when such benefits could be achieved at acceptable cost. It should not be given in situations where possible harm outweighs any possible benefit. Within a group of patients for whom intensive care is considered, the likely outcome of such care is a major consideration. The panel suggested use of a simple scale for prospective patients:
1. Expected to survive, potentially recoverable (a good chance).
2. Prognosis uncertain.
3. Death probable shortly, whatever is done.
4. Death apparently imminent.
   In view of public expectations of what medicine can achieve, the panel recommended that in the United Kingdom intensive care should be considered for the first two of these categories, if the costs are not prohibitive. This would seem to be a practical and pragmatic, rather

than an ethical, approach; it recognizes that facilities are limited. The panel also suggested that it may be appropriate to admit potential organ donors (that is, those patients who have suffered brain-stem death or are expected to do so) because procedures such as mechanical ventilation are required to keep the organs in good condition. The treatment of many patients with heart, lung or kidney failure depends on the supply of organs for transplantation. In cases of brain death, the recommended policy is to provide optimal care for the dying patient until it is agreed that further therapy is useless, when there is a shift in emphasis from prolonging life to maintaining organ viability. There is a more difficult problem with those whose prognosis is uncertain, but we try always to give patients the benefit of the doubt; and in the absence of reliable data on which to base decisions, such patients should also be treated in the ICU.

Patients whose death is probable shortly whatever is done provide a different dilemma. It is often possible to produce temporary improvement to allow time for relatives and the medical team to come to terms with the inevitability of death. It is in these cases that the question of benefit to the patient is most difficult to assess, and here also that we have to consider the question of the continued use of ICU resources which might ensure the survival of other patients.

### Assessing benefit

Doctors and others often disagree about the probability of benefit to a given patient, and about the degree of benefit that should be regarded as worthwhile. In such cases, benefit should be assessed not merely in terms of survival but in terms of the survivors' quality of life.

The concept of benefit has been the subject of numerous interpretations. The King's Fund panel considered the question of whose judgement of benefit should prevail in doubtful cases. The Hippocratic (and also the British and American Medical Associations') view is that the physician should benefit the patient according to his or her ability and judgement. This statement is paternalistic in that it depends solely on the doctor's subjective judgement, and makes no provision for the autonomy of the patient. In extreme cases it has even been evoked in defence of bizarre experimental therapy as well as forced feeding and unnecessarily invasive treatment.

The panel preferred the following formulation: 'The physician should benefit the patient according to the most objective judgements available unless the patient expresses a competent and informed wish for an alternative course.'

One problem about admission to intensive care units is the fact that resources are limited. Moreover, intensive care treatment is very expensive because of the high staffing levels and expensive technology that are required. It seems appallingly callous to ask if it is financially worthwhile to keep patients alive; but it must be remembered that in intensive care we have the potential ability to continue treatment, and in effect to prolong the process of dying, even in cases where there is little prospect for recovery.

In our own unit we have sometimes admitted patients we know to be dying only because the unit has better staffing levels than anywhere else in the hospital. A young man was brought into our unit suffering from 94 per cent burns (that is, 94 per cent of the surface of his body was burnt) following an automobile accident. He and his three friends had been driving home from a party when their car hit a lorry. The three friends died instantly, but he was dragged out of the flames and rushed to hospital. It was clear that he could not survive: with burns of this extent and degree of severity there is no way to find enough skin for the necessary grafting. He simply came to the intensive care unit for nursing support. I shall long remember the smell of burning flesh given off by this man. He was treated with morphia and passed away within 24 hours of his admission to our unit.

## Health-care policy

Doctors today face not only a challenge to their clinical autonomy – that is, the right to make clinical decisions without reference to anyone but the patient – but also a growing move to minimize their role in formulating health-care policy and financing. It is an unfortunate fact that the cost of health care accelerates at a rate unacceptable to legislators, unions and businesses. Physicians need to understand the desire to control costs. The spectre of admission to intensive care being controlled by administrators has arisen recently because intensive care is expensive, and it could be argued that it is unfair to spend so much on so small a number of patients. Economic decision-making by our physicians would seem preferable to the menace of inviting non-physicians to make what are plainly clinical decisions however they may be camouflaged as efforts at cost control or quality assurance. In fact, the British NHS reforms do offer the opportunity for units to control their own budgets.

There is great pressure today to reduce costs by what may be termed 'quicker and sicker' discharges. 'Quality control' may be a code term for cost containment and reduction. It is possible that recent efforts at peer review organization and audit may not only be failing to save money but actually adding to the costs of the administration of health care. Various interested parties have looked at factors which could be used as guidelines for admission – or, to put it another way, as justification for limiting admission of certain groups of patients to intensive care. Levinsky* recently examined age as one such justification. He questioned the acceptability of limitations on health care for the elderly, and challenged the suggestion that medical research and development of health care aimed at extending life should not be funded. This brings up the spectre of patient selection.

In American society there is an emphasis on youth as a value in itself. There is a suggestion, too, that physicians may be extending life as a goal in itself, beyond the persistence of any spark of humanity and against the will of the patient and family. This concern about technology for its own sake is especially focused on the elderly. Levinsky noted that, 'Medical care that extends life devoid of human qualities should not be undertaken – but this principle should be applied to patients of all ages, not only the elderly.' If rationing is instituted we should allocate resources according to the probability that the patient will benefit, rather than his or her age. In any case, it has been pointed out that in the United States the economic benefit of rationing intensive care high technology for the aged would be small, as such expenditures account for only 3.5 per cent of Medicare expenditure.

In 1973 Medicare, the health insurance cover given to elderly people in the United States, assumed financial responsibility for dialysis. Before 1973 dialysis patients were predominantly white, middle class and with high education status; often such patients were selected by a committee. Since 1973 distribution of patients receiving dialysis for endstage kidney failure much more closely reflects the demographic make-up of the American population. In times of selection, those who know how to 'work the system' receive treatment preferentially; the poor, ignorant and disadvantaged bear the brunt of resource limitation.

* Levinsky, N., 'Age as a criterion for rationing health care', *New England Journal of Medicine* (1990), 322, 1813-15.

The whole idea of selection of patients is abhorrent and at its extreme point conjures images of an ICU doctor conniving with his infamous colleague, Mengele, who selected patients for life or death in the Nazi concentration camps. This, of course, is an unfair comparison: patients coming to the ICU are desperately sick and the technology and skill deployed in intensive care may represent the last valiant attempt to save somebody doomed by uncontrollable disease. Most patients who have been treated in an ICU (and their families) would want such treatment again, even if it gave them only one extra month of life.

Medical ethicists have agonized over the question of the allocation of resources to intensive care, and indeed to medicine in general. This is illustrated by the discussions of the Appleton Consensus,* which considered the question of allocation of scarce resources. They noted that it may not be feasible to offer everything medically possible to all patients. They suggested that, in determining priorities with scarcity of health resources, some concepts play critical roles:

1. Justice – universal access to an acceptable, decent minimum of basic health care.
2. What is acceptable varies with society and time. Judgements are required about health-care needs.
3. If society decides on health-care provision for all, resources must be so directed.
4. Medical decision-making must emphasize cost effectiveness so the burden of universal access may be reduced.
5. The market place cannot be the sole determinant of priorities.

The Appleton Consensus ethicists went on to argue that guidelines must be laid down to establish the limits and priorities for life-sustaining treatment. The procedures used to establish such limits must be perceived to be open

* Stanley, J.M., 'The Appleton Consensus: suggested international guidelines for decisions to forgo medical treatment', *Journal of Medical Ethics* (1989), 15 (3), 129-36.

and fair, taking into account cost effectiveness. They suggested further that society must be willing to adjust to such expectations. If the institutional limits imply that physicians must deny care to some patients, physicians have an especially strict obligation to weigh burdens and benefits in selecting patients for care and treatment. Patients do not have a right to treatment which has no reasonable expectation of benefit, but treatment denied on social grounds must not be disguised as a medical decision. Physicians must protest if treatment is withheld improperly, and private purchase of treatment must be restricted if it impinges on general access to scarce resources.

### Treating the elderly

There are situations where admission to intensive care is mandatory – for instance, following major cardiac surgery, when the blood circulation is frequently very unstable and can be monitored and controlled properly only in the intensive care unit. On the other hand there is often pressure to prolong intensive care unjustifiably in situations where heroic operations have been carried out but have proved unsuccessful. We see many aged patients in our ICU and it is certainly not our policy to deny admission. An example was Mrs J.D., aged 89, who presented in the casualty department with obstruction of her bowels. This type of mechanical problem can never be resolved medically. It was decided to operate, and it was found that part of the large bowel was perforated and that intestinal contents were soiling her abdomen. Within 24 hours she died of persisting shock.

Should this patient have been operated on at all? It is quite possible that the staff on duty when she came in did not have the seniority or experience (or indeed courage) to decide against a possibly life-saving procedure. In the event the procedure itself probably did not add significantly to her suffering. In many cases of abdominal catastrophe, the only certain way of diagnosis and cure is by operation, but the doctor must always give the patient the benefit of the doubt.

Another woman, also in her 80s, was admitted to the hospital with acute abdominal pain. After some resuscitation – that is, stabilization of her fluid balance and blood pressure – an operation was carried out and it was found that she had cancer of the rectum, which fortunately did not appear to be too advanced. Post-operatively she required intensive care treatment with artificial ventilation. Her progress was very slow; at times it seemed she could not recover because of the multiplicity of her problems. Antibiotics and blood pressure support were withdrawn after consultations with the surgeons, and soon after she suffered kidney failure. Then, to our surprise, she gradually improved. Further antibiotics and physio-therapy were given as we began to have doubts over our pessimistic assessment of her chances. Our dilemmas increased when we discovered that she had been housebound for months before this acute crisis, with a very poor quality of life. Theoretically she had a surgically removable and curable cancer. However, after three or four weeks on the ventilator she could not be weaned off it, and eventually we had to fashion a tracheostomy – an opening in her trachea or main air passage in the throat through which her ventilation improved, so that she breathed satisfactorily unaided. She went to the ward, but died there a few weeks later.

Again, one might question whether the original operation should have been carried out. But a doctor's first duty is to relieve pain, and this seemed to be the only way that this could be achieved. The more serious question is, was the reduction of treatment justifiable? At that time the situation seemed hopeless because she had many organ system failures.

## Limiting factors

Criteria for admission to intensive care units vary within each institution. Many things influence whether or not a patient is admitted to intensive care, including such non-clinical factors as bed numbers and the availability of nurses. A controversial case was that of an elderly man whose arteries to the bowel were diseased. This had resulted in perforation of the bowel, with the inevitable release of faecal content into the abdomen. The patient arrived at a time when the nursing staff in the intensive care unit were at the end of their tether owing to reduced numbers and demoralization caused by increasing workloads. They did not feel that they could continue to provide a safe service if they accepted an additional patient. In addition to the technological aspects of their work, the nurses are faced with the constant emotional burden of dealing with severely ill patients and with their relatives. The surgeon in this case insisted that the operation should go ahead, arguing that there was no possibility that the patient could be transferred to another institution or have his operation delayed. The nurses reached a point of mutiny. Following the operation, the patient required ventilation for only some 48 hours before he was returned to the ordinary ward – rather earlier than we would have liked, but it was felt that some intensive care was perhaps better than none at all.

As I mentioned in Chapter 2, Professor Vincent in his survey on European attitudes towards ethical problems in intensive-care medicine reported that a shortage of ICU beds is common and that admissions to intensive care are generally limited by the number of beds. This was a factor in 57 per cent of the units which he surveyed. On the other hand, two-thirds of the intensivists who responded said that they had admitted patients with no hope of survival for more than a few weeks.

It has been suggested that entitlement to intensive care could be determined by an index directly proportional to the probability of successful outcome, quality and length of life remaining and inversely related to the cost required to achieve therapeutic success. The idea is interesting in theory – but how could one determine the quality and length of life remaining with any precision? I have had no personal experience of such an index nor do I know if it has been tried in practice.

This approach raises many ethical problems. It is well known that in the United Kingdom there is a serious shortage of dialysis facilities. As I am a kidney specialist as well as an intensivist I have frequently had to face the problem of patient selection. Many of the patients whom I see with chronic kidney failure are elderly, but some renal replacement units are not anxious to take them on because, first, such patients have a limited prognosis, and second, they may prove a burden on the dialysis unit because they will require more nursing and medical care, so reducing that available for others.

Unquestionably their lives will be prolonged by dialysis, and it is for this reason that I try to make sure they are properly placed on chronic renal failure treatment programmes. Sometimes my colleagues in the dialysis unit chide me on the grounds that I push them to accept sickly patients on to a programme for which I do not take personal responsibility. Obviously, if one could be sure the patient would not benefit by the treatment, it would be wrong to refer them. But this is a very difficult judgement to make. Often the patients are mentally confused and, particularly in elderly people, the question arises as to whether such confusion is something unconnected with renal failure and is an irreversible disability, or is the result of acute poisoning caused by their kidneys' inability to excrete normal waste products.

A problematic case was a woman of 67 who presented, mentally confused, and in renal failure. She proved difficult to treat because of her lack of co-operation. Once it was clear that her kidney failure was not going to be reversible, she was referred to a chronic dialysis unit. There, too, she proved a problem. She was so confused and frightened that at one stage she hid in a cupboard on the ward. In the United Kingdom many older patients, including this patient, are treated by chronic ambulatory peritoneal dialysis (CAPD), in which a tube is inserted into the abdominal cavity and dialysis fluid is run in and out.

I later met one of this lady's children and was pleased to hear how well she is coping with her dialysis. She is fortunate, particularly in these days. She has five loving children who take it in turns to look after her and carry out the dialysis for her at home. At the time of writing no complications have occurred and she has not needed re-hospitalization. Thus she is not a burden on the renal unit and her life has been prolonged, which is her wish and that of her family. And although her mental confusion remains, it seems to be improving and she is able to cook for her extended family! The problem of shortage of dialysis facilities in the UK mirrors the shortage of intensive care facilities. Both these deficiencies are due to the underfunding of health care in the UK as compared to other Western countries.

### Improving admission procedures

We would like to see patients come earlier to intensive care. If problems such as fluid depletion, infection, or circulatory failure are corrected early the patient's prospects may be better. Often patients arrive only when they are in urgent need of mechanical ventilation, by which time the seeds of multiple organ system failure may have already been sown.

Sometimes these problems are not easy. A man of 71 was admitted to hospital having suffered a couple of episodes of angina some 10 years before. He came in this time after having suffered 20 minutes of chest pain and was treated for a further heart attack. He seemed to be doing well. He had an episode where he was said to be overbreathing. It was known that he had had an anxiety neurosis while serving in the army. He required treatment with a urinary catheter which distressed both him and his family. They had been devotees of alternative medicine, particularly homeopathy, and were not happy in the ward. On the sixth day of his admission the patient and his wife both requested discharge. At that time he was continuing to overbreathe, was described as being tremulous, and showed some signs of incipient heart failure.

The staff on duty in the ward tried hard to dissuade him from this course, but in fact it was only the late hour that prevented the patient from leaving. That night the medical officer on call was summoned because the patient's condition had greatly deteriorated. He was grossly breathless owing to acute failure of the left side of his heart. No intensive care bed was available at that time.

Over the next few hours his condition got worse. Five hours later it was possible to admit him to intensive care, where he was given the full panoply of treatment, with drugs to support his blood pressure and basic monitoring, and so on; but within four hours he was dead from a cardiac arrest. It is tempting to think that had he come to intensive care earlier he might have been saved. The case, however, illustrates the fact that some patients have their own strongly held views on the situation. It may well have been that he would have refused the chance of earlier intensive care treatment.

There is growing concern, inside and outside the NHS, about the fate of patients who are refused admission to intensive care. In fact, they are often given some lesser form of intensive care by the doctor and nurse especially assigned to them on the ward, but without the mechanical support and special skills available in the intensive care unit. We do everything possible to avoid this less than satisfactory alternative, which is why we now have a written policy for admission to the unit. This is a set of guidelines on how patients should be admitted to ensure smooth running of the unit and to maintain fair access to all patients.

Sometimes patients are referred to a particular hospital because of the special skills available there. These specialized units may require the support of intensive care if problems arise, and, again, this may be difficult if the ICU is full. At my hospital we have a special unit for laser therapy, and some time ago a patient was referred for laser treatment of intractable gastrointestinal bleeding when the intensive care unit was already fully stretched. It was felt that the laser method of controlling the bleeding was preferable because the patient lived in a nursing home and weighed 100 kg (about 16 stone), suggesting that she was unable to look after herself and that the risks of an operation were greatly increased by her obesity and attendant poor health. Unfortunately, the attempt at laser therapy failed. We were faced with a dilemma. If she came to surgery she would inevitably require ventilation and prolonged intensive care support. We decided that as she had been sent to us from another institution for a particular procedure which no longer seemed appropriate, the right course of action was to return her to her referring hospital. In a way this avoided the ethical dilemma of whether or not to operate on her. In fact, of course, we merely passed the problem back to the referring institution.

Another tragic case was treated first in a neighbouring hospital. A 63-year-old Vietnamese refugee was treated for an acute abdominal catastrophe. At surgery he was found to have a perforation of the intestinal wall and there were free faeces present in the abdominal cavity. A colostomy, opening the bowel to the abdomen wall, was fashioned, but no ICU bed was available at the hospital. He was treated first in their recovery area and then in a corridor next to the intensive care unit. Later he was referred to us and presented very short of breath with severe hypoxia (lack of oxygen) and very low blood pressure. He had what is called adult respiratory distress syndrome (ARDS); another complication was the fact that his white cell count, which usually rises in response to infection, was actually low. He developed multiple organ system failure and required haemofiltration (circulation of the blood through a filter, as in dialysis) as well as drugs to raise his blood pressure to support his circulation and mechanical ventilation. Five days later he developed an abscess under the diaphragm muscle that separates the lung and abdominal cavity. We struggled with him for a month until his condition finally deteriorated and he died.

It is recognized that patients suffering from a lack of oxygen around the time of an operation do badly. Further, two of the aims of intensive care are to optimize blood flow and oxygen delivery. Clearly, in the hassle to try to find a bed for this poor man, neither of these aims was achieved. We were never able to make up for the damage which occurred in those first few hours after operation.

Another aspect of the problem of admission to intensive care units is the fact that major surgical operations are planned on the understanding that the patient will be nursed in the intensive care unit for the first day or so after leaving the operating theatre. If the intensive care beds are blocked by long-stay patients or, as is commonly the case, by inadequate resources for intensive care, then patients awaiting surgery are put at risk. Today some patients stay in intensive care or high dependency wards because there is no bed elsewhere for them in other part of the hospital. The stark fact is that far more patients die while *awaiting* cardiac surgery than those who are victims of surgical problems. It has been shown in surveys of the use of organs donated for transplantation that a significant factor is the availability or otherwise of intensive care facilities. There are many well documented instances of the wastage of donor organs – which almost certainly has resulted in the death of the intended recipients – owing to there being no intensive care facilities available at the critical time.

I do not deny the need to examine, regularly and objectively, the criteria for admission to intensive care. But the painful ethical dilemmas that ICUs face up to every day in the United Kingdom result first and foremost from inadequate provision of intensive care resources. There is abundant data to show how the United Kingdom lags behind in the provision of such resources, as indeed it does in many other areas of modern medicine.

There is also a need for adequate data collection and analysis to show the benefits of intensive care for particular groups of patients. The effects and value of the various techniques of intensive care need in some cases to be elaborated in order to support the demand for more facilities. They would also help resolve the question of who should be treated in intensive care.

# 5

# Intensive Care: When to Stop

One of the ethical objections levelled at intensive care is that it prolongs the process of dying rather than saves life. The fact is that it is extremely difficult in the ICU to know *when* to stop trying to save life. The ideal, obviously, is for the patient to recover. But what of the patient who struggles on week after week without evidence of real progress? Are there any ethical guidelines as to how long this battle should continue? To put it another way, is it *ever* ethical to withdraw treatment? The problem is particularly acute in patients who do not have an ostensibly fatal, malignant disease or who are relatively young. Sometimes family pressures or pressure from colleagues may dictate continuing treatment beyond the limits that we think are reasonable. Long, and in retrospect futile, struggles are notoriously undertaken with national leaders. The late Emperor Hirohito of Japan was effectively treated in intensive care for about four months before he finally succumbed. Similarly, some years ago the late Marshal Tito of Yugoslavia had his life prolonged over and above what one might reasonably have expected in a man of his age. The same occurred in the case of the late dictator of Spain, General Franco, possibly to allow time to decide the question of his political succession.

Some of the patients described below also had political

connections, but this was a matter of chance and I do not think it impinged on the decisions of their treatment: they all had prolonged stays in intensive care because of the nature of their illness, not because of who they were. These cases show just how hard it is to know when to give up the struggle.

A first cousin to the ruler of one of the Persian Gulf emirates had a very long history of duodenal ulcer which seemed to be resistant to most forms of treatment. The time had come for him to have an operation, which in view of his degree and duration of suffering was entirely reasonable. A standard operation was performed by an eminent surgeon. Three days later he became very ill and was transferred to a hospital with better intensive care facilities.

The diagnosis of perforation of an abdominal organ was made. He had developed a stress ulcer in his stomach following the original procedure. It is recognized that patients in the severely ill post-operative period can develop acute ulceration of the stomach which may have nothing to do with their underlying condition; and that was thought to be the case here. Post-operatively he bled: on one occasion he required 28 units of blood within a 24-hour period. Numerous experts were consulted and X-rays of the arteries to the intestines were repeatedly made to find the cause of the bleeding.

He also developed evidence of septicaemia, respiratory failure and kidney failure requiring artificial ventilation and treatment with haemofiltration. During most of the remainder of his course in hospital he was only semi-conscious. He required a total of nine abdominal operations. The condition of the abdominal cavity became increasingly disorganized and the operations became more and more technically difficult. He was a strong and brave man who at the time of this illness was only 56 years old. He did respond when the situation was brought under control by getting the right mix of blood products, antibiotics and nutrition and at times he was able to speak to us. This made his continuing deterioration all the more distressing for all concerned.

He had numerous other problems including skin infections, ulceration of the eye and jaundice. The continuing major problem was the fact that the intra-abdominal situation was never fully under control, despite all our attempts at investigation and treatment, both medically and surgically. It was a tribute to the sophistication of techniques available that we were able to keep him alive by ventilation, dialysis and parenteral nutrition for 90 days. Eventually he again developed overwhelming bleeding, and by then he showed evidence that his brain was no longer functioning. Neurologists were consulted, but regrettably it was no longer felt that there was any point in trying to keep him going.

His management in a private intensive care unit meant that the consultants did the routine work themselves because of the absence of skilled junior intensive care staff in such private hospitals. Often the experienced resident is more capable than his senior colleague, certainly at some of the technical aspects of management, and in this and other ways thinly medically staffed private clinics may be hazardous for the patient.

This patient had a potentially recoverable condition. The fact that he was treated in the private sector had little bearing on his management as I am sure we would have carried out the same treatment in our unit at University College Hospital. It was unfortunate that we were never totally able to control the bleeding for long enough to enable full recovery. It was tantalizing for all of us because at times we felt confident that we would succeed. It was this conviction that we could pull him through his devastating illness that encouraged us to continue for 90 days. The financial cost was irrelevant.

### Treating young people

Young people present a specially poignant challenge. A 14-year-old boy developed acute leukaemia. He was treated with anti-cancer chemotherapy and developed pneumonia, which required artificial ventilation. He became unconscious and ventilation was continued for some 10 days without any signs of recovery. Eventually he died in spite of all our measures. It might be thought that the position should have been recognized as hopeless. But nevertheless we continued to try to control the infection, hoping the chemotherapy would be effective in controlling the leukaemia.

I had occasion to discuss the tragedy with his father some six months later. He felt that every moment of his son's life had been worthwhile, and had he been given the opportunity he would still be sitting by his son's ventilator, even though he felt his chance of recovery was remote. In this case treatment was not withdrawn or reduced in any way, but unfortunately nature took its course.

A 12-year-old diabetic girl had a back operation in a private clinic. In such cases, one can be assured of excellent hotel service. In the United Kingdom at the time of writing, one can also be assured that the surgeon of one's choice will do the operation, together with his chosen anaesthetist. Unfortunately, none of the private clinics in London currently has more than a skeleton resident medical staff. This is in contrast to the situation in the impoverished state sector, where at least in the major teaching hospitals there is a reliable network of well-trained junior staff capable of dealing with any emergency.

This little girl's problems began over the weekend following her operation. She developed signs of a catastrophic leakage of bowel contents into the abdomen and became obviously septic and ill. Following the weekend, when she was seen by her surgeon again, she was transferred in shock to an intensive care bed in an NHS hospital as a private patient.

For the next four weeks the staff struggled against her increasing array of failing organ systems, using ventilation and haemofiltration, and finally treating her with a form of extracorporeal membrane oxygenation, a kind of artificial lung, because she was not able to achieve adequate oxygenation through her own lungs. Inevitably, she died.

During this course a variety of operations had been done as abdominal complications had occurred. Again the staff were faced with a 12-year-old girl, and while there was any possibility of survival, the dedicated intensivists continued the struggle. Whether this was cost-effective, rational or an appropriate use of resources is another question.

### Diagnostic problems

Another long struggle took place in the final illness of a 61-year-old African politician, one of the architects of the struggle for independence of a former colony of Portugal. He fell ill at home in Africa and came to Portugal, whence he was transferred to London. His illness presented initially with fever and then he developed enlargement of the liver and spleen and anaemia. The question of some bone marrow disease was raised and a diagnosis of hairy-cell leukaemia, which is usually fatal, was suggested. In addition, tuberculosis was diagnosed (it is quite common to develop tuberculosis in immuno-suppressed states such as one has with leukaemia or with its chemotherapeutic treatment).

When he was admitted to our intensive care unit he was very ill, in respiratory failure, with pneumonia. He was treated with interferon (a hugely expensive anti-viral drug), numerous diagnostic procedures including lung and liver biopsies were carried out, and there was persistent doubt and discussion over the diagnosis. At one stage, a month after his admission, he was much improved and able to get out of bed with minimal support to his ventilation. However, he then developed further bleeding, which was possibly compounded by the haemofiltration, which requires the use of blood anti-coagulants. He bled from various parts of his body, including his gut. He suffered further deterioration of his lungs, he was given drugs to support his circulation, but in spite of this he developed persistently low blood pressure, and on the 56th day of his admission to intensive care he died.

This patient's primary problem was a disease of his bone marrow; it is likely that the diagnosis of hairy-cell leukaemia was correct, although this was disputed by some. In addition, he had tuberculosis, fungal infections, pneumonia, bleeding, problems with his gastrointestinal tract, circulatory failure and kidney failure. Our difficulty, in terms of deciding if and when to stop intensive care, was that on the 30th day of his admission he was out of bed, alert and requiring only minimal support. It may be that we underestimated the severity of his underlying disease process, which I think was the reason for his fatal outcome. The fact is, it was difficult to be certain of his diagnosis during life. It unfortunately is often the case that things become clearer only when it is too late. I do not think we would have been justified in stopping his treatment in any way, even though in retrospect we seem to have persisted for an inordinately long time. If a similar case occurs again it is difficult to see how we could have done otherwise.

In all the patients described in this chapter there was reason to hope for recovery almost up to the very end. They illustrate how difficult it is to lay down rules as to how long treatment should be continued in intensive care;

in particular, they show the difficulty of making generalizations from specific cases. Our policy is to continue while there is any hope at all of recovery, in spite of the pressures we experience and the limits on finance and facilities.

# 6

# Withholding Intensive Care

One of the most difficult clinical dilemmas we face in intensive care is the question of withholding treatment from patients. Can this ever be justified?

Professor Vincent in his survey of European intensivists (see page 11) discussed the problems of withholding and withdrawing life support. Although there may be no ethical distinction between withdrawing and withholding treatment, the majority of intensivists felt less comfortable with withdrawal. This may be emotional, reflecting the reluctance of doctors to take the positive step of stopping what may be life-saving (or at least death-delaying) treatment. The effect of withholding treatment may be the same, but the patient does not usually remain in the unit as a visible cause of concern, guilt and doubt. Also, by withholding treatment the intensivist does not have to face and comfort the family. Of the 239 respondents to Professor Vincent's survey, in patients judged to have no real chance of recovery it was common to withhold or withdraw sophisticated therapy (83 per cent of the group said they were prepared to withhold, whereas only 63 per cent were prepared to countenance withdrawal of therapy).

The problem raised by withholding therapy can be illustrated by a number of the cases I discussed in earlier chapters. On one occasion intensive care treatment was almost withheld because of shortage of staff and worries that, if we committed the patient to intensive care, it would be much more difficult to withdraw treatment later, rather than refuse admission in the first place. The patient in question was a man in his 80s who had undergone a recent operation for ischaemic bowel (disease caused by poor blood supply). This particular condition carries a very high mortality rate, which is naturally a cause of concern and sometimes pessimism in the unit.

He came back to the hospital with a further bout of abdominal pain two months later. His circulation was compromised, as shown by the fact that his kidney function was impaired, and he was taken to the intensive care unit to resuscitate him prior to further surgery, as he presented with signs of an acute abdomen necessitating an urgent operation.

The intensive care staff examined the patient in detail because of the anxieties of taking on an elderly, probably hopeless long-term case at a time when both facilities and nurses were under pressure. Fortunately, it was concluded that there was no alternative but to operate. However, we knew that if further ischaemic bowel disease was found, we would be reluctant to take on long-term intensive care in a man of such advanced years who had undergone recent surgery. The prognosis of acute abdominal conditions in people of his age is poor, and would be especially so if he had a recurrence of his ischaemic bowel problem. But should intensive care be denied, as a matter of policy, to people who are old and whose prognosis is poor?

The operation went ahead after the patient had been resuscitated in intensive care. It turned out that he had acute appendicitis, which was treated surgically, and made a good recovery without the need for intensive care after the operation. Yet the intensive care staff had been quite justifiably concerned that they might have to take on a long-term patient with a very poor prognosis.

This case illustrates the dangers of possibly inappropriate intervention being undertaken: if too doctrinaire an attitude had prevailed we would have denied the patient his operation and his chance of recovery. Intensive care *before* surgery contributed greatly to the successful outcome and prevented the need for prolonged and probably ineffective post-operative treatment. Good preparation for surgery in order to stabilize vital functions may be one of the most effective forms of intensive care.

A clear-cut case of treatment withheld occurred in the sad case of a 20-year-old Ghanaian boy who fell in love while in England. His feelings were not reciprocated, and he felt that he needed to make a gesture and unfortunately decided to drink car-battery fluid, which consists of concentrated sulphuric acid. He drank some 400 ml, which is far above the recognized lethal dose, and the acid burnt holes in his diaphragm, stomach and intestines. He underwent emergency surgery and his condition appeared to stabilize. However, the surgeons told us that he was left with only a very small amount of intestine, that it was likely that the areas burned by the acid would fall apart, but that it was simply not worthwhile to attempt further surgery. It was very eerie talking to this doomed young man, who was conscious for long periods of his illness.

We sought further surgical opinions as to whether there was any possibility of saving him but we were repeatedly assured that such attempts would be futile. After a few days he developed signs of peritonitis. This inflammation of the lining of the abdominal cavity was presumably caused by disintegration of the bowel wall with leakage of faecal fluid. Before he died he told us that he regretted his suicide gesture which had gone so horribly wrong. In view of the decision that his condition was both inoperable and unsalvageable, the full gamut of intensive care was withheld from him but he was kept comfortable.

## AIDS and alcoholism

Sometimes treatment is withheld from groups of patients as a result of hospital policy. A common example of such policy is found in those hospitals where patients with AIDS, developing severe pneumonias as a result of their drastically lowered resistance to infection, are not admitted to intensive care. This policy reflects the fact that the results of treating such infections, especially second bouts of infection of this type, are very poor. However, first bouts of pneumocystis pneumonias can quite often be cured. (Pneumocystis is an organism that becomes a cause of serious infection only in people whose resistance is very low.) The results of treating pneumocystis infection are improving. I believe a blanket policy of excluding all patients with a particular diagnosis from intensive care is worrying and very probably wrong.

It may be that staff in intensive care units are worried about treating patients with AIDS. However, the danger to staff is perhaps greater from patients who have undiagnosed AIDS or are carriers of the HIV virus. Sometimes AIDS patients specify that they do not wish to have intensive care treatment. On the other hand, we must be very careful to ensure that patients are not excluded from intensive care treatment as a result of prejudice.

Another illustration of the ease with which treatment might be withheld occurred with a 29-year-old homeless alcoholic, who had been drinking five bottles of Martini a day. He came in with abdominal pain, initially thought to be appendicitis but subsequently shown to be caused by tuberculosis. He was extremely ill and developed kidney, liver and respiratory failure. On top of everything else, he was highly uncooperative. Nevertheless, he was curable. The intensive care unit was full. It is rarely possible to cure alcoholics of their addiction, and their life survival is limited. The dilemma was: should we transfer someone, perhaps more socially responsible or stable, out of intensive care to make room for him? This problem was compounded by the knowledge that one of the causes for his kidney failure (at that moment his most immediate problem) was overdosage of streptomycin, prescribed for his life-threatening tuberculosis. We eventually started some further supportive but less adequate treatment in the ward without transfer to the intensive care unit, and he made a slow recovery. His underlying problems remain but treatment was not denied. We hope, probably vainly, that he will not return to his alcoholism.

Another reason for withholding intensive care inappropriately is simple ignorance of treatment possibilities on the part of physicians caring for severely ill patients in the wards.

Intensive care, then, is withheld on a number of grounds. Strictly speaking, the only grounds that are not ethically dubious to at least some extent are if the patient specifically refuses it or if it is certain that it will be medically useless. It seems to me unacceptable to withhold intensive care on grounds of prejudice against patients with specific diseases or antisocial habits. All too often the problem of withholding treatment arises because there are simply not enough intensive care beds and/or nurses to offer treatment to all who could benefit, underlining again the need to expand intensive care facilities in the United Kingdom.

# 7

# Withdrawing Intensive Care

Some ICU consultants have argued that the question of whether clinicians should switch off life-support machines should not be swept under the carpet but bravely addressed. Those holding this view have suggested that ICU patients who do not recover after four or five days typically become septic and develop multiple organ system failure, at which point clinicians should consider treatment withdrawal. It is suggested that prolonged intensive care may merely prolong suffering, waste resources and ultimately achieve nothing. This is an extreme view, and not one to which I subscribe. Nonetheless, particularly in these times of cost consciousness, it is one that is being heard.

In Professor Vincent's survey, 63 per cent of 239 European intensivists felt that withdrawal of intensive care therapy should be done. This, of course, is a higher percentage than those who are prepared to countenance euthanasia. Although there is debate as to the distinction between withdrawal of treatment and euthanasia, there is a clear difference in intent. Withdrawal of treatment is usually done when it is felt that further treatment is useless, both medically and ethically, in the face of overwhelming disease. Euthanasia implies a positive act to end life: it is a destructive act of commission, albeit with the connivance of the patient.

In practice, rather than equipment being switched off, the usual way in which treatment is withdrawn is by the failure to institute further treatment when new complications arise in a patient who is already mortally sick with a number of organ system failures. Sometimes justification for withdrawal of treatment leads to speculation as to the purpose of medical treatment itself. According to some, medical purpose is related to the improvement of the quality of life, which may be unattainable in very damaged individuals. This does not necessarily justify the withdrawal of minimal support to keep patients alive. Assessment of the quality of life is highly subjective and one could call into question the ethical authority of those who based their treatment programmes on value judgements of this kind. In any case the presumption that someone has a poor quality of life in no way invalidates their right to survive.

### The Quinlan and Cruzan cases

In the United States the question of treatment withdrawal has been extensively discussed and the law has evolved as the result of a series of cases. Karen Ann Quinlan was a young girl who lay in coma for years. Hers was the first case in which an American court – the Supreme Court of New Jersey in 1976 – condoned the removal of life-sustaining medical care from a permanently incompetent adult. The case came to court because the family wanted active treatment support to be withdrawn. The physicians refused, as the law was not clear. The court ordered Karen to be removed from the ventilator if the family, the physicians and the hospital ethics committee agreed. In the absence of information from the patient personally, the doctors and the family had the right to make the decision to withdraw life support.

The court clearly implied that in such situations the family's wishes could override the physicians' concerns. Put another way, 'substituted judgement could be made for the incompetent adult'. In their judgement the court in the Quinlan decision examined the 'reasonable possibility of return to cognitive and sapient life as distinguished from ... biological vegetative existence'. The Quinlan case is undoubtedly important for what it decided: that there comes a point beyond which a doctor is no longer under a duty to persist with forms of treatment which can be described as pointless. The rights of the patient, the family and the position of the doctor in this respect were discussed. The decision has been regarded as a major advance in the development of humane and sensitive medical law.

Ironically, when the ventilator was removed, Karen Quinlan was able to breathe on her own and lived on for 10 years in a persistent vegetative state, unable to respond to her surroundings, until she died. Her case has become a byword for the rights of patients and their families.

The question of the rights of patients, particularly in relation to withdrawal or refusal of treatment as compared to the role of the doctors and the courts, has been extensively explored in the United States with a series of cases underlined by the celebrated Nancy Cruzan case of 1990. The problem with Nancy Cruzan was that she had been in a comatose state since 1983 following an automobile accident, requiring tube feeding and minimal medications but no other mechanical assistance to continue to survive at a very basic level. Her parents believed she would not want to 'live like a vegetable' on the basis of her own statement that she would not want to continue to live if she could not be at least halfway normal.

A judge authorized that tube feeding be discontinued, but the doctors looking after her were unhappy with this decision and challenged it. Eventually the Missouri Supreme Court reversed the decision on the grounds that no one could decide on Nancy's behalf. They took the view that she maintained her most basic functions, and they upheld a biological definition of life rather than one involving more complex abilities. The court ruled that the state had a legitimate interest in preserving life, regardless of its quality. The state required clear and convincing evidence that the patient herself would not want treatment to continue life in such circumstances, otherwise (the court reasoned) incompetent patients with all manner of handicaps might find the state (or their families) seeking to terminate their lives.

The final arbiter of legal issues in the United States is the Supreme Court in Washington, which can overrule decisions by the individual states' supreme court. Nancy's parents appealed to the U.S. Supreme Court, the court's first case involving the right to refuse life-sustaining treatment. The question at issue was the right of surrogate decision makers to act on behalf of previously competent patients. The concern was that this was literally a matter of life and death and that abuses could occur if incompetent patients did not have loved ones available as surrogate decision makers. The Supreme Court split five to four in favour of the Missouri Supreme Court, upholding the view that the state's prime interest and duty is to protect life.

Following the Supreme Court decision a judge heard further new evidence which achieved the clear and convincing standard of proof required by the Missouri legislation that Nancy Cruzan would not have wanted her life to be maintained in her present state, and permitted the discontinuation of life-support treatment. Nancy Cruzan died in December 1990.

This episode has caused considerable soul-searching among bioethicists, and a group of them issued a statement commenting on the U.S. Supreme Court decision in the Cruzan case.*

---

* Annas, D.J., et al, 'Bioethicists' statement on the U.S. Supreme Court's Cruzan decision', *New England Journal of Medicine* (1990), 323, 686-7.

First, the Supreme Court affirmed the right of competent patients to refuse life-sustaining treatment.

Second, the Court did not treat the forgoing of artificial nutrition and hydration differently from the forgoing of other forms of medical treatment.

Third, the holding in the Cruzan case was only that the state of Missouri could require the continued treatment of a patient in a persistent vegetative state unless there was 'clear and convincing evidence' that she had explicitly authorized the termination of treatment before losing the capacity to make decisions.

Fourth, the Court did not require that other states adopt Missouri's rigorous standard of proof.

Fifth, the Cruzan decision does not alter the laws, ethical standards or clinical practice permitting the forgoing of life-sustaining treatment that have evolved in the USA since the Quinlan case in 1976.

They commented further that

Physicians should continue to be guided by the ethics of the medical profession and accepted clinical processes concerning the withdrawal of life-sustaining treatment, unless and until these are challenged or changed by law.

One of the consequences of the Cruzan case in the United States was increased awareness and use of the so-called 'living will' (this is discussed more fully in Chapter 10). Basically, in the living will the patient gives directives in advance on the use or withdrawal of life-sustaining treatment should he/she become incapable of making decisions themself. There are various ways in which treatment may be withdrawn. Usually it is by the deliberate decision not to institute further escalations of therapy. In the United Kingdom the legal position about withdrawal of treatment is not clear. The question of withdrawal of treatment will be illustrated by some of our cases, where such withdrawal has taken place hopefully with the agreement of all concerned.

Sometimes relatives request withdrawal of treatment from a patient whom they consider to be 'suffering'. In fact, it is most unlikely the patient is suffering himself, but clearly the sight of patients in intensive care is very distressing for their visitors, who are often appalled by the proliferation of tubes and machines applied to their loved ones. My reasons for saying that patients do not suffer in intensive care are, first, that it is general policy to keep them very well sedated and, second, that when one asks patients who have survived prolonged periods in intensive care to describe their experiences, these have almost always been forgotten.

It is obviously difficult to be dogmatic on this question. It may happen that when patients are being weaned from dependence on ventilators it is important that they are awake, and there may then be periods of confusion with some distress.

### Irretrievable damage

An example of a patient whose treatment was withdrawn was a man of 71 who had leukaemia which appeared to be under fairly good control when he presented as an acute emergency complaining of headache. This was shortly followed by cardiac arrest. Resuscitation was undertaken before he came into hospital. A CT scan showed that he had had an extensive subarachnoid haemorrhage, causing pressure and damage to the brain. When this evidence of haemorrhage was found, support for him was withdrawn on the grounds that damage to the brain was so extensive that he had no chance of recovery. He required drugs to maintain his blood pressure, and a ventilator to support his breathing, and there was no evidence of any conscious brain activity. It was thought justifiable not to add any further measures to support him. Accordingly no new drugs or blood or increase in drug dosage was given and the patient died shortly afterwards. There was objective evidence here of devastating brain damage in a man already ill with a fatal disease.

Sometimes questions arise with patients who have severe infection complicating their alcoholism. One is concerned as to how hard one should try with people who seem irretrievably damaged. The guideline must be that if there is any serious possibility of recovery, everything must be done. Unfortunately, there are all too many derelict alcoholic patients in the inner city area which we serve.

A 47-year-old man came in to us in a collapsed, confused state. He had severe diarrhoea and vomiting, possibly caused by an infection (alcoholics, like other people who are addicted to various agents, have a lowered resistance to infection). In the course of his illness his heart stopped. This was restarted. He required mechanical ventilation, and although we were able to wean him from the ventilator after a few days, he was sent down to the ward in a semi-conscious state. It seemed very unlikely that he could survive for a prolonged period.

Our aim is always to remove ventilatory support from patients as quickly as possible; but I am always concerned as to whether early discharge of such patients to the wards is not in fact a way of withdrawing support, because the level of staffing in the wards is not sufficient to provide optimal care. Unfortunately there is tremendous pressure on the intensive care facilities and such decisions may be inevitable within the constraints of our resources.

## AIDS: a special problem

The question of treatment withdrawal had to be considered in the case of a patient with AIDS. He presented to the casualty department after taking an overdose. He had a cardiac arrest there and was resuscitated and brought up to the intensive care unit. It was then that we discovered he was a patient with AIDS who had previously had pneumocystis pneumonia. He had recovered from this, but he had recently suffered a recurrence and he decided that he did not want to live any longer. His partner had recently died of AIDS. This information was not available to the doctors in the casualty department, but had been written down in a note which a friend brought in to the hospital a few days after his admission.

The problem in intensive care was whether it was justifiable to withdraw treatment in view of the patient's own wishes. One shrinks from the very idea of switching off ventilators. This man, besides requiring artificial ventilation, needed drugs to support his blood pressure and antibiotics for his pneumonia. His condition stabilized, but we then became aware of the fact that he had been depressed because of the death of his partner. He was aware that he himself was suffering now from advanced AIDS with the recurrence of his chest infection. The problem was, first, should we treat him effectively against his known wishes? He had stated that he did not want to fight on in view of his advancing AIDS. Second, we felt he was unlikely to recover. The question arose as to whether and how it was justifiable to withdraw his treatment. Eventually, in consultation with experts on his condition, we decided to keep him breathing with room air only instead of giving him high-concentration oxygen. He was kept in intensive care until he died after five or six days. Our dilemma was whether or not to respect the patient's wishes, given the exacerbation of the emotional factors arising from his illness. Would it have been ethically preferable to switch off the ventilator rather than to ventilate him ineffectually as was done here? We are always concerned to maintain sedation to ensure that the patient does not suffer. This patient did not want intensive care, but were we right to withdraw it from him?

Many authorities would debate this. One should always presume that patients want to survive, and even in patients with AIDS the right course of action is to start resuscitation. The ethical position on treatment withdrawal is still unclear, and even less clear is the question as to how such withdrawal may reasonably be undertaken. In this case we had good evidence that we were acting in line with the patient's recorded wishes.

## Long-haul treatments

Sometimes treatment is withdrawn at the end of a long and unsuccessful struggle to save a patient's life. A 58-year-old man, with a background of heart disease, chronic obstructive airways disease and tuberculosis, developed inflammatory damage to many of his organs, vasculitis. For a long time this was undiagnosed. He presented in his final illness with weight loss. Eventually the position became all too clear when he bled through the rectum and an arteriogram, or X-ray of the artery, revealed no blood supply to the gut owing to blockage of an artery. This particular condition has a mortality rate of over 80 per cent in patients who also have any generalized disease.

Following the diagnosis, his large bowel was removed. He required 15 units of blood for this operation; he continued to bleed, needing another 25 units in the next 24 hours, and a further operation was done. A third operation was carried out when bleeding continued. As a result of this he was left with only 20 cm of gut. However, the bleeding persisted. By the time he had had 56 units of blood with continuing haemorrhage, it was decided not to transfuse him further on the grounds that, with only a fraction of diseased gut remaining, it was most unlikely that he could survive, and that in any case he would require treatment with continued parenteral nutrition intravenously if survival were possible. He had multiple organ system failure affecting his lungs, kidneys and heart. The position was discussed with the family, who agreed that his prognosis was hopeless. No more antibiotics were given as well as no more blood, and a few hours later he died. The question arose as to whether his treatment should not have been stopped earlier.

*Persistent vegetative state*

The final case of treatment withdrawal also took place long after the patient left intensive care. It concerned a 17-year-old boy. His case is perhaps the most worrying of this worrying group. The history was that he tried to pull a soft-drink bottle out of a vending machine. Somehow he managed to pull the whole machine on to his head and suffered irreversible brain damage. When he arrived in hospital his heart had stopped, but he was successfully resuscitated. He was treated on the ventilator for a few weeks in intensive care until he was able to breathe on his own. He required persistent treatment with anti-convulsant drugs because of his epileptic fits. He did not regain consciousness. Examination of his nervous system demonstrated little remaining brain function. It was felt that he had severe and irreversible brain damage, although since he could breathe unaided he could not be classified as brain dead.

This young man was in a persistent vegetative state, able to maintain his breathing and other vital functions without mechanical aids but unable to respond in any meaningful way to stimuli. In addition, we needed to give him anticonvulsant drugs to control his fits. There were efforts to remove these drugs to assess his level of consciousness, but the fact that he was not brain dead made the decisions in his case even more difficult than those others described above.

The question arose as to how heavily he should be supported. At one stage it was discussed with his mother whether or not he should be fed. She visited him daily and took an extremely keen interest in his welfare, and she rapidly came to the conclusion that we should not feed him. It was a very difficult decision for the doctors to accept, and it is questionable whether it should have been accepted. Eventually, four months after the boy's injury, her wishes prevailed. Feeding was withdrawn but fluids were continued and, after four months in a twilight state between life and death, he died. Interestingly, this lady later spoke in a BBC radio programme about euthanasia, which she supports.

The problem of withdrawing treatment is particularly acute in patients, like this boy, who are in a persistent vegetative state. Although able to breathe and maintain their circulation without assistance, they are unable to move in any purposeful way or react in a coordinated manner to stimuli, and their level of awareness is extremely limited. Occasionally, people who have been described as vegetative may recover. In a reported series of 500 patients who were described as being in this state, only three regained independence. In an extreme case, a professor who had suffered brain injury due to lack of oxygen was able to resume his duties at his university and to all appearances returned entirely to normal. This patient had come perilously close to having his life support withdrawn and it was only the persistence of his family which ensured that treatment continued.

The difficulty when withdrawing treatment from patients in the persistent vegetative state is that they may survive for months or even years. One patient in this condition survived for more than 37 years. This is the other side of the coin of treatment withdrawal. In patients in a persistent vegetative state, the decision to withdraw treatment does not usually directly concern the intensive care unit, since they are treated in other areas of the hospital. However, one is inevitably concerned that the decision to send them down to the ward, inescapable with our current pressures on intensive care beds, may be condemning these people to death or to years of essentially meaningless existence.

The persistent vegetative state can also be defined as a stable condition in which the patient has no cognitive function and is incapable of experiencing pain and suffering. It follows that withdrawal of feeding and/or hydration might be acceptable to some authorities, who would argue that this does not result in cruel or violent death. In the case of the boy who was in a persistent vegetative state following the soft-drink vending machine accident, after he was discharged from intensive care the decision to withdraw feeding was taken with the consent of his physicians but at the instigation of his mother. Hydration was maintained.

I continue to be troubled by this decision. The caring mother's wishes were respected, but I have grave doubts as to whether it is ethically defensible to deny food to a patient. This, of course, is a point for debate; not everyone would agree with my view. It seems to me that there is a clear ethical as well as clinical distinction between the case of a patient who is in a persistent vegetative state and one who is brain dead. For the brain dead patient there is no doubt about the outcome; for a patient in a persistent vegetative state, the prognosis is far less clear cut. In the case of this boy we were influenced by the caring mother's attitude and her insistence that feeding be withdrawn. It is a decision that still causes us anxiety because we could not know how much, if anything, the patient in a persistent vegetative state is able to experience and appreciate. The boy was treated with full support for at least three months before the feed was withdrawn. There had been absolutely no sign of recovery, which convinced us that the possibility of improvement was extremely unlikely; and this, together with evidence of extensive brain damage on CT scans, allowed us after much heart-searching to support the mother's pleading.

A 79-year-old man suffered a heart attack near our hospital. Passers by naturally rush to the aid of such people, who are brought into the hospital with very little evidence of heart activity because attempts at cardiac resuscitation outside hospital are rarely totally successful. This patient spent three days in intensive care and we were only slowly able to wean him from ventilatory support. He had developed complete paralysis of one side of his body, but he continued in a semi-conscious state for a further month in the ward, until he developed pneumonia. The question of withdrawal of treatment arose only when he was transferred to the ward. The dilemma of treatment withdrawal in this case did not directly concern the intensive care staff – except that his treatment in the ICU enabled the man to survive and, thus, for the problem of treatment withdrawal to arise.

His brother visited him daily and was very concerned about his welfare. The patient was unable to communicate in any meaningful way or to respond to pain or other stimuli in a purposeful or organized fashion. We asked for and received neurological opinions and they confirmed our view that there was no hope of any significant recovery. We therefore decided, when he developed pneumonia, that this should not be actively treated with antibiotics – but did not discuss this question with his brother. Does this indicate medical paternalism? The patient was in a persistent vegetative state. Is it ethical for doctors to decide against life-prolonging treatment for such a patient without even consulting the next-of-kin? Are we allocating medical resources at the bedside, or the ward round? Clearly doctors have to make decisions: the question is whether they should have the only or final word on such matters. In the United States the position is quite different from that in the UK.

The decision to withdraw treatment is one of the hardest tasks for an intensive care doctor. Whom should he ask or tell? How should it be done? We often try to wean unconscious, damaged patients from ventilator dependence, knowing that when they return to the ward they may well die of pneumonia. Should we explain to the family the full implications of our actions? Strictly speaking, responsibility rests with the team of doctors that cares for the patient in the ward. We know the staffing levels in many wards do not allow patient abnormalities or crises – for example, inhalation of secretions – to be detected and corrected as quickly as in the intensive care unit. In the United States these matters are discussed freely and openly, and they should be in the United Kingdom, too.

It is always important to establish good rapport and mutual confidence with the patient's relatives. If the decision to withdraw treatment has been made on medical grounds – and indeed on humane grounds, for the family more than anyone else – then there is no point in escalating or even continuing active treatment. But the full implications of this must be explained and understood. The emphasis of management is then changed to ensuring the patient's comfort and tranquillity. Specific treatments such as haemofiltration can then be withdrawn. More difficult are decisions not to give antibiotics when the patient develops an infection, or to withdraw them. In fact, withdrawal of antibiotics may be in the best interests of the patient, as many courses of antibiotics are prolonged unnecessarily and they occasionally give rise to fevers themselves. Fluids are prescribed to ensure that there is some maintenance of body water but the constituents of the fluid and salt replacement need not be adjusted to match the worsening body chemistry.

It has been suggested that such measures are euthanasia in disguise. One cannot pretend that this situation is easy to handle. Relatives may well harbour lingering doubts as to whether everything possible has been done and whether it is really right that the doctors appear to have given up. Equally, the staff may feel guilty about stopping treatment – they may have become emotionally entangled in the patient's troubles and the family's problems. On the other hand, there may be a sense of relief that the patient is being allowed to gently fade away and that the perceived suffering of the patient and, more particularly, his family, will not continue.

The problem in some patients failing to improve in intensive care is the development of multiple organ system failure and the inability to respond to increasing treatment. Although perhaps mortally ill, they are quite distinct from patients in a persistent vegetative state. The difficulty in such cases is to know when it is permissible to give up trying to cure the patient, to know for certain that nothing more is possible.

I must emphasize that life-saving treatment is withheld or withdrawn relatively infrequently from patients in intensive care. However, such decisions precipitate about half of all deaths in such circumstances. The patients are usually unable to take part in the decision, but obviously it is important for physicians and relatives to agree on the limitation of care. Often the family, emotionally drained by many days' vigil at the bedside watching increasing efforts meet with diminishing success, accept the necessity to withdraw treatment even before the doctors are ready to admit defeat.

# 8

# Resuscitation:
# Decisions & Dilemmas

One of the reasons for the development of intensive care units was the introduction and refinement of the techniques of cardiopulmonary resuscitation (CPR). This has meant that it is now possible to re-start the heart in patients who have suffered a cardiac arrest and also to support those patients whose breathing has suddenly stopped. Techniques have been disseminated, perhaps not widely enough, to members of the general public. What is required if the heart stops is to support the circulation by massaging the heart through the chest wall – external cardiac massage, and at the same time to maintain respiration by breathing into the patient's lungs.

These techniques have a long history. Perhaps the first recorded case of cardiopulmonary resuscitation was performed by the prophet Elisha on the son of the Shunamite woman (II Kings iv, 34). Nowadays, following cardiac arrest, it may be necessary to give the heart an electric shock to re-start it or to reinstate an adequate heart rhythm to enable proper circulation of blood to take place.

Patients who have a cardiac arrest in hospital are obviously best placed to receive adequate resuscitation. Outside hospital one has to choose one's passers by in selecting where to have a cardiac arrest. Our hospital is situated near three major railway stations, and we see at least one patient a month admitted with a cardiac arrest after being resuscitated in one of these stations by a passing physician.

The success of resuscitation depends on a number of factors, including the expertise of the personnel; perhaps the most important factor is the length of delay between the actual arrest and the institution of resuscitation. One of the problems is to know how long one should persist in what appear to be vain attempts to resuscitate. This is important, not only in the immediate period after the arrest, but also in patients who are in intensive care following cardiac arrest and appear to be making slow progress.

A case in point was a lady aged 67 who was admitted to the intensive care unit following a cardiac arrest. She remained in shock, needing continuous infusions of drugs to support her blood pressure for three or four days. While in the intensive care unit she had another cardiac arrest and again was in prolonged shock. She eventually made a complete recovery and could return home. During her time in intensive care, because of her profoundly depressed levels of consciousness and circulation, she showed evidence of acute kidney failure, and, more importantly, she required ventilatory support for one week. In spite of all these problems, thanks to the benefit of energetic support, she survived to go home. Her total stay in the intensive care unit was 12 days and at times her very survival was in doubt.

It is remarkable that a life-threatening abnormality of heart rhythm – the usual cause for cardiac arrest – can occur without there being very extensive damage to the heart tissues themselves, so that if the abnormality can be controlled the patient's long-term outlook is actually very good.

Unfortunately the situation of patients who have

cardiac arrest in addition to some other illness is often much worse. A 62-year-old woman was admitted having taken an overdose of alcohol together with Heminevrin, a drug used to aid withdrawal from alcohol dependence. It is basically a sedative and unfortunately it, too, can be abused, as in this case. This patient had a cardiac arrest. She required artificial ventilation for a period of some 48 hours. Then she was sent down to the wards to an uncertain future. She was still unable to cough or breathe properly and it seemed likely that she would develop a chest infection which could prove fatal.

The question arises again and again with such patients: how far should one's efforts go? Should we not have kept this woman longer in intensive care? We manage patients over the period when they require mechanical support and try not to pass judgement or advice on their subsequent course in the ward. It is not our job to make value judgements on people but to resuscitate them and, in a sense, to pass on the problem to somebody else. Is this really the best way to go about things?

Quite often patients who have cardiac arrests underline the difficulty of withdrawing treatment when all seems futile and lost. A 70-year-old suffered a cardiac arrest outside our hospital. He was resuscitated by medically trained personnel who happened to be passing and was brought into the casualty department, where it was apparent that he needed ventilation. He had persistently low blood pressure, although his heart beat spontaneously. While in intensive care he showed no evidence of recovery and required increasing doses of drugs to support his blood pressure. Eventually he appeared to become resistant to the effects of these drugs. Further supporting measures were not added and he died after some 36 hours.

He was treated in the intensive care unit until his pupils became fixed and dilated; they did not respond to any stimuli, and this is one of the criteria of brain death. Were

our efforts misplaced? Would it have been right to
withdraw treatment sooner? This kind of result is
unfortunately common in patients suffering cardiac arrest
outside hospital. Survival is often dependent on the
degree of damage that occurs to other parts of the body at
the time of the cardiac arrest, rather than to the degree of
damage to the heart itself. There is a need for more people,
including the general public, to learn efficient techniques
of cardipulmonary resuscitation to improve the outlook
for people suffering cardiac arrest. Better transport to
hospital would help, too.

## The Ethics of 'DNR'

In some countries and cities ambulances are equipped to
go out to cases of cardiac arrest, and even helicopters have
been used for this purpose. Often the deciding factor
against survival in patients with cardiac arrest is the fact
that they may suffer extensive irreversible brain damage
during the time when they have no blood circulation. One
of the patients mentioned above showed signs of brain
death on admission to the intensive care unit; others have
shown only a very low level of consciousness, being able
to breathe but capable of little else.

There is obviously an ethical imperative to attempt
cardiac resuscitation of patients in whom the heart has
stopped – unless, of course, this is against the patient's
known wishes, or the arrest occurs as a result of some
incurable illness such as terminal cancer. This raises the
question of the place and significance of 'Do not
resuscitate' orders. One could argue that if too much time
has elapsed between cardiac arrest and the arrival of
medical assistance, resuscitation should not be started as
inevitably the patient will, even at best, be incapable of
leading an independent existence. Yet it is very difficult
for doctors deliberately to forgo trying to help, and the

ethical ramifications of such an approach are considerable. The ethical dilemma arises in how to handle these patients. Should they have full support forever? What exactly *is* full support? Is one justified, for instance, in making a decision to withhold antibiotics, with or without discussions with the relatives?

Most patients in whom 'Do not resuscitate' (DNR) orders are contemplated or given are patients severely brain damaged by haemodynamic instability, or patients judged to have no real chance of recovery, such as those with terminal cancer. In the United States attempts have been made to legislate ethics and there have been discussions of the consequences of codifying the process of medical decision-making, particularly the withholding of life-sustaining therapy, including cardiopulmonary resuscitation. It is a fact that CPR has been withheld and that DNR orders have been given by doctors for many years. These problems are discussed by McClung and Kamer.* Active consultation with the family, but obviously not with the patient, is required only for acts of commission such as disconnecting treatment with a ventilator, a measure taken only after the fullest possible consideration.

The whole question of DNR orders in the United States was sparked off in 1981 by the death of a woman in a Queen's Hospital (New York) intensive care unit, following which there was an enquiry because the institution did not offer cardiopulmonary resuscitation. New York State passed a law that every patient who has not consented to a DNR order is assumed to have consented to CPR.

In my view this kind of legislation leads to more resuscitation rather than less and in many cases this resuscitation is inappropriate. A case came to my

---

* McClung, J.A. and Kamer, R.S., 'Legislating Ethics: implications of New York's Do Not Resuscitate law', *New England Journal of Medicine*, (1990) 323, 270-72.

knowledge which occurred following the passing of this law in which a woman of 95 stopped breathing following a massive stroke. Resuscitation was continued for 3½ hours until her only relative could get to the hospital on a snowy night to consent to withdrawal of resuscitation. (I discuss later the problem of obtaining consent when patients are no longer capable of making decisions.) Difficulties arise if the presumption of consent to CPR is taken to mandate CPR in every case. However, often the fear of legal consequences forces medically inappropriate decisions. In fact, according to McClung and Kamer, patients are involved in DNR decisions in only 13-28 per cent of cases.

The proper aim of written or legislated policy on resuscitation should be that it is the physician's duty to provide adequate information for patients and appropriate surrogates so that full, meaningful consultation about these vital decisions can occur. Professor Vincent commented on DNR orders in his survey of policy and attitudes of European intensivists. He found that they are usually verbal, although about two-thirds of his respondents thought that they should be written. Only 7 per cent of his survey group discussed DNR with the patient. Clearly it is impossible with most patients, but 25 per cent of his respondents felt that such orders should be discussed. A majority, 57 per cent, involved the family in these discussions. Interestingly, families were consulted more often if the intensivist was older than 40 or considered himself religious.

A large majority of intensivists apply DNR orders to avoid futile therapy for refractory circulatory shock, or prolonged downhill or irreversible disease with permanent brain damage. The worry, of course, is how certain one can be about prognosis, but there is clear evidence that the longer patients remain in intensive care without evidence of cerebral activity, and with continuing deterioration, the worse are the chances of any kind of recovery.

In our unit we do try to write down DNR decisions when these have been reached. We have frequent discussions with the family, whom we keep fully informed. In those cases where we feel resuscitation would be futile – if the patient has been in septic shock for several days and then his heart has stopped – the chances of any kind of recovery of cardiac function, let alone recovery of the whole person, are as good as zero. We do not baldly say to people that we are instituting a DNR order. We explain that, in spite of all our efforts, the patient has not recovered and we have reached a point where further additional treatments will not be instituted because we consider they would be futile. We are, of course, always open to the family asking for a second opinion if they are unwilling to accept this decision. In the vast majority of cases, when they have seen that we have striven for a long time with skill and dedication, they are more able to face the inevitable and accept the loss of their loved one.

There have been attempts to lay down policy about cardiopulmonary resuscitation (CPR), and blanket policy always attracts criticism. Cases have been quoted where patients with terminal cancer have been resuscitated. Equally some patients who, although very elderly, were otherwise viable have not been resuscitated for reversible conditions because of an absence of clear written guidelines on this important question. Sometimes, particularly in the United States, symbolic Hollywood-style attempts at resuscitation are made when everything is done in slow motion to satisfy the need to be seen to be doing the right thing. In studies of CPR, 60 per cent of patients were successfully resuscitated – but only 3 per cent went home. This underlines the need to define the term 'success' in resuscitation. It would seem that such resuscitation is inappropriate in patients whose lives are naturally drawing to a close due to terminal illness. A further instance where a DNR order might be justified is where CPR is not anticipated to be of medical benefit, either because it cannot succeed or because of the patient's previously poor quality of life. Equally, patients whose quality of life would be poor after resuscitation might be candidates for a DNR order; but this is clearly more dubious, as are all ethical decisions based on perceived 'quality of life'.

Implicit in DNR orders is a judgement of the quality of life. Is it right that the quality of life is determined by the ability to move and speak and that, therefore, anyone who has a poor quality of life should not be treated for a life-threatening condition? Cases have been cited in the literature in which a DNR decision has been made regarding mute, quadriplegic patients. But such people are able to interact with their environment and even to appreciate jokes.

The other question raised by the issue of the DNR order is the definition of resuscitation. Does this include the giving of fluids and nutrition to patients in a persistent vegetative state? If one established a DNR order, could these treatments be withdrawn? There is a 'hard' ethical line here because of the historic symbolic significance of food and water. There appears to be a natural line between DNR and starving someone to death. Interestingly, as we saw in the previous chapter, nutrition and hydration were not regarded differently from other forms of treatment by the United States Supreme Court in the Cruzan case. The whole issue bristles with ethical traps.

The application of DNR orders, then, has sometimes led to paradoxical results, including an increase in inappropriate resuscitation in institutions where a DNR policy is mandatory. If a patient arrives and such a policy has not yet been laid down, medical staff, particularly juniors on duty at night, and especially if the 'hand-over' of patients between duty doctors has not been explicit, may feel compelled to carry out resuscitation, even on inappropriate terminal patients.

In the United States there has been a study describing the effects of discussing DNR orders with a group of patients with malignant disease. These discussions took place before the patients were in a terminal state. All were either distressed or depressed by the discussion, which added to their anxiety, or they suppressed all memory of the discussions.*

Rarely, if ever, are DNR orders discussed with patients in intensive care in the United Kingdom. The vast majority of the sickest patients could not comprehend them or give answers because of their illness, but as is our policy, DNR orders are discussed with the family. In these discussions the doctor needs to give clear guidance as to what he feels the prognosis is and what chance there would be of resuscitation being successful. Usually when sick intensive care patients suffer cardiac arrest it is the result of the continued irreversible deterioration in their underlying condition, making resuscitation and DNR irrelevant.

It has been suggested that CPR inflicts humiliation and suffering on the dying. Elderly people who are demented, with conditions such as Alzheimer's disease, would seem to be suitable cases for DNR orders. Some enthusiasts for DNR orders have put forward the suggestion that useless prolongation of life should be an offence! There is genuine concern in the public mind about ill people not being allowed to die: but the concept of life not being worth living is clearly subjective, and in any case should be applied by an individual only to himself, not to anyone else.

The conflict between CPR and the place of DNR orders is a good example of the ethical dilemmas of intensive care. In a sense CPR was the godfather of intensive care and the life-saving techniques of CPR remain one of its cornerstones. If CPR is only partly successful and leaves

---

* Schade, S.G. and Muslin, H., 'Do not resuscitate decisions: discussions with patients', *Journal of Medical Ethics*, (1989) 15, 186-90.

the patient in a persistent vegetative state, which many people may feel is a fate worse than death, then it may precipitate the heart-searching that inevitably accompanies the question of treatment withdrawal. Another consequence of the development of CPR is the expectation that anyone who dies needs CPR – which is clearly absurd. But in hospital, unless there is a written DNR order, CPR may automatically and inappropriately be attempted. DNR orders can be given when medically it is certain that CPR would be futile. The question of consent to DNR is also very thorny; it is recognized that patients have a right not to consent to CPR, but obtaining a patient's consent for either CPR or DNR may be emotionally distressing at a time when they are already suffering and may be incapable of giving a competent answer. The place of relatives and other surrogates to give consent is a further source of doubt and debate.

Finally the poor results of out-of-hospital CPR in many places underscores the need for better training of the public in resuscitation techniques and more effective organization of emergency services.

# 9

# Autonomy

Autonomy has become a cardinal principle in modern secular medical ethics. It implies that individuals have a sovereign right to determine their own destinies, unfettered by external moral influences or strictures. This is in spite of the fact that for the greater part of human history religion has been seen as the foundation of morality. In Dostoevsky's words, 'If God did not exist, all would be permitted'. It was Immanuel Kant who insisted that being moral cannot be a matter of submission to an external authority but must be something that we impose on ourselves in what he called autonomy. This fits with the idea that morality is a matter of individual choice. But there can be both law and morality without the constraint of religious tradition. This led to the idea that patients have the right to determine what happens with their lives and, in some extreme cases, to end them at their will.

The principle of autonomy is enshrined in the Appleton Consensus, in which international guidelines for decisions to forgo medical treatment were suggested. As the first principle for the ethics of physicians providing medical treatment, they declare the principle of autonomy to mean that physicians must respect others' autonomy and choices.*

* Stanley, J.M., 'The Appleton Consensus', *Journal of Medical Ethics* (1989), 15 (3), 129-36.

A further point is that treatment carried out in a public institution may have an element of coercion and external authority. The possibility arises, at least theoretically, of interference in a person's bodily integrity and individual liberty.

## Limits to autonomy

Problems obviously arise when a competent patient refuses treatment which the physician believes to be in the patient's best interests. The physician should explore the reasons for the refusal and correct any misunderstandings, but he should not impose treatment if the patient rejects it (even if the treatment is potentially life-prolonging), and should explore alternatives which may be acceptable to the patient. Even when a specific treatment is refused by the patient, the physician and the hospital have the obligation to continue to offer supportive care and treatment to relieve pain and suffering.

Requests for futile treatment – that is, treatment either with a low probability of success or that would leave the patient with a poor quality of life – are not binding on the doctor, who should explain all treatment options and his or her opinion regarding each. If a physician has a conscientious objection to a requested treatment, he is not obliged to provide it. But if the patient wishes, the physician should transfer his or her care to another physician of the patient's choice.

These ethical problems of the limits of patients' autonomy were discussed by McClung and Kamer.* They referred to the policy of the Beth Israel Hospital (Boston) published in 1976 by Rabkin, Gillerman and Rice which

---

* McClung, J.A., and Kamer, R.S., 'Legislating Ethics', *New England Journal of Medicine*, (1990) 323, 270-72.

allowed patients to refuse CPR regardless of the medical situation. A surrogate could consent to a DNR order on behalf of patients judged incapable of giving consent themselves.

It is often impossible to honour the patient's autonomy if he or she is admitted as an unconscious emergency. Doctors will always give the patient the benefit of the doubt and resuscitate rather than waste time trying to find out what are the patient's wishes and directives, if any. Doctors rightly prefer to err on the side of life. And although people may theorize about not wanting resuscitation or intensive care, they may feel very differently if the need for such treatment suddenly arises. While information should be shared with patients, I am doubtful whether the full gory details need to be told to everyone, as shown by the study, cited in the previous chapter, of the effects of discussing DNR orders. Moreover, prognosis is perhaps the area where doctors are most fallible.

The question also arises as to which of a patient's relatives, if any, is empowered to make decisions for him or her. Occasionally relatives disagree as to what is in the patient's best interest. The doctors need to take a firm, educated, informed line, having presented the facts.

We have had a number of cases which illustrate the difficulties with this question of autonomy and the dilemmas that arise from it. A man of 57, known to be mentally defective following meningitis as a child, had a past history of alcohol abuse and had been unable to cope since his mother had died some three years previously. He was known to the social services, who visited his home and found him to be in an appallingly neglected condition. He had not seen any relatives for some two years and seemed to be confused and living in isolation. He was malnourished and had lost weight; he had difficulty with recent memory, and was thought to be vulnerable and at risk because on several occasions he had wandered away from his home and not been able to find his way back.

He was admitted to the hospital as an emergency after being found lying under or close to a steamroller throughout a January night. When he came in he was unkempt, unshaven and hypothermic, with a tender abdomen. He gave a past history of a duodenal ulcer. He was extensively investigated and thought to have alcoholic dementia; he also had a gastrocolic fistula which had developed after his ulcer operation years ago. The psychiatrist recommended that he be placed in an institution or a hostel for such dependent people. However, it was felt that in order for him to find a place in such a hostel he would need to have the fistula repaired, as it caused severe diarrhoea, which he found very difficult to control and made him socially unacceptable. The situation was explained to him and it was suggested strongly that he consent to an operation, but he refused. It was felt that he understood what was being suggested to him. There seemed to be an imperative to find suitable accommodation for him and this meant him undergoing the operation. Eventually he did give his consent. The operation proved complicated, the fistula was undone, the bowel repaired. Unfortunately the surgical connections that were made leaked after a few days and he went into shock because of the peritonitis caused by the release of intestinal contents into the abdominal cavity.

He developed septicaemia and as a result developed difficulties in his blood-clotting system and required support with ventilation, maintenance of his blood pressure, transfusions, replacement of blood products, antibiotics and vitamins. He also required intravenous feeding, developed increasing failure of his lungs and required a tracheostomy to facilitate his breathing, and became jaundiced. Eventually, in spite of further attempts to repair the damage, faecal fluid was found to be leaking from his abdominal wound. Twenty-three days after the ill-fated operation he died.

Should he not have had the operation? Could we have withdrawn support earlier in view of the multiple organ system failure? If so, at what stage? Instead we battled on till the inevitable end. Did we wrongly overrule his autonomy by pressing and repeating the request for surgery, which his instinct told him to refuse? He had initially declined to have the operation, which was advised because he had distressing symptoms and the surgical treatment represented a way to get him placed in an institution. Were we interfering with his liberty? But was there any feasible alternative course of action?

### Autonomy and self-abuse

Another aspect of the question of autonomy was presented by a man who is a regular patient of our ICU. He has long-standing chronic bronchitis and has been admitted with exacerbations three times, requiring ventilation of at least five days on each occasion. After his second visit he was observed to be smoking shortly after he had been weaned from the ventilator. This type of character is a natural target for the ire of health-care workers, particularly the ex-smokers among them, who resent the fact that shortly after they have made great efforts to relieve exacerbation of a smoking-related disease, the patient is going back to the same habit. However, whether this resentment is justifiable is much more debatable.

There is an unequivocal relationship between smoking and the development of chronic bronchitis. The question arises as to whether doctors would be justified in refusing to treat patients who persist in their harmful habits. In my opinion they would not. As it happened, this particular patient did well after his third episode of ventilation and is now able to carry on with his normal activities, including walking out of doors. He tells me he has even stopped smoking.

A similar problem was presented by the sad case of an alcoholic who had started his career as an engineer. We came to know him and see him increasingly in the last months of his life. He died when he was 46 years old. He was a regular attender at the casualty department of the hospital, usually arriving with a variety of problems. On one occasion he had a fractured skull after having been beaten up. On another occasion he came in in a psychotic state, showing features of depression as well as the bizarre psychosis seen in alcoholics and associated with confabulation, Korsakoff's Psychosis, in which patients invent fantastic imaginary events. This was associated with another alcohol-related condition, Wernicke's Encephalopathy, which is characterized by weakness and paralysis of some of the nerves in the area of the head. He then developed a pancreatic mass and we wondered whether he had cancer, but this was never proven.

Interestingly he was able to come off alcohol at times, but he had various chronic problems, including homelessness, related to his longstanding alcoholism, and these problems soon drove him back to drink every time he stopped. Finally he had a series of bouts of vomiting blood. These were shown to be caused by bleeding from oesophageal varices, varicose veins in the gullet. Attempts were made to control this bleeding, first of all by injecting the bleeding points and then by applying pressure through what is called a Sengstaken tube. On this penultimate admission he told us that he wanted the bleeding stopped but was not prepared to stop drinking. He returned shortly afterwards, once again with a torrential haemorrhage from his oesophagus, and it was then decided to perform an oesophageal transection, which involves cutting across the oesophagus and sewing it together to block the veins. Following this operation he again required intensive care. He deteriorated steadily, his lungs stopped working and increasingly high concentrations of oxygen were required for gas exchange.

He needed drugs to support his blood pressure, and then his kidneys failed. The question arose as to how hard we should try to save him. He had shown no ability to withdraw from the alcohol for any significant period of time, and his prognosis if he continued to drink was hopeless.

One might argue that the operation should not have been carried out in the first place, but it is very difficult to stand by and allow somebody to die of haemorrhage. Equally, one could argue that it is unethical not to try everything possible to save the life of a 46-year-old who does not have cancer – though the prognosis of cirrhosis of the liver is in every way as bad as that of many types of cancer. On the other hand, it would seem reasonable to expect patients to cooperate with medical treatment and this man's record showed that this was impossible. One could argue that a patient has a duty to his medical advisers just as much as the medical advisers have a duty to the patient. Eventually, he was ventilated and was given antibiotics for his chest infection as well as drugs to support the blood pressure; but he died five days after his transection operation, despite maximal intensive care.

Another variation on the patient autonomy theme was represented by a man who had bacterial endocarditis (infection of the heart valves) and was progressing well with antibiotic injections. He begged to be let out for a few hours to see to some business outside the hospital. He went off with his cannula in place in his vein ready for the next injection, but failed to return. We discovered the next day that he had returned to Scotland and it seemed doubtful whether he was going to complete his course of treatment. We tried to contact his old doctor and the police, but we were not optimistic about his return. He did come back six days later in a far worse state and needing replacement of his heart valves now destroyed by untreated, uncontrolled infection.

Patients with anorexia nervosa represent another

extreme of the autonomy spectrum. A question that arises with these patients is whether it is ethical to force-feed them. On occasion they have been put under psychiatric section, permitting this to be done. Such an action is undoubtedly well-intentioned, but it is ethically dubious and of debatable effectiveness. Rabbi Jonathan Sacks in his 1990 Reith Lecture summed up the situation with regard to autonomy: 'acts are freely chosen: consequences are dealt with by the State. Governments, therefore hospitals, are there to treat AIDS, child abuse, homelessness and addiction, but not to disseminate a morality that might reduce them in the first place'.

### AIDS: autonomy and confidentiality

I have seen few patients with AIDS coming through intensive care, but guidelines on their ICU management may be needed in view of the predictions that the numbers of AIDS patients will increase. A 46-year-old man was admitted to our unit with a high fever. It was known that he was an alcoholic and sometimes abused drugs. Initially, homosexuals were the major group of patients in the United Kingdom infected with AIDS, followed by those abusing intravenous drugs, and latterly there has been a slowly increasing incidence among heterosexuals. This man had a prolonged illness; he was found to have meningitis, which was treated successfully. It then became apparent that he had cirrhosis of the liver and he developed kidney failure.

It is not permitted as a routine in the United Kingdom at present to carry out tests for AIDS, looking for the human immunodeficiency virus (HIV) without consent; but in situations where it may be important for the patient's welfare to know this, the test may be done. In this case the patient was found to be HIV positive and his blood was infectious. There is a difference between carriage of the virus and having the full-blown syndrome, which was not present here. It is recognized that other than sexual intercourse, transmission of the virus is quite difficult, though unfortunately some people have acquired this syndrome previously through contaminated blood transfusions. Nowadays this risk is negligible because all blood donors are screened for the HIV in Great Britain.

Our nurses were extremely worried about the possibility of handling blood which was HIV positive when the possibility of dialysis treatment for his kidney failure arose (this requires an extra circulation of blood outside the body). We were also concerned as to whether the virus could contaminate the machinery. However, there are systems for carrying out dialysis using entirely disposable equipment. This patient's kidney failure was treated, but he died of other infections. Nonetheless, the case illustrated another dilemma. The reaction of the staff to such patients varies, but this cannot be allowed to influence clinical decisions.

A further variant on the patient autonomy theme came in another alcoholic aged 64 who came into hospital with a chest infection. He was agorophobic and also phobic of doctors. His pneumonia was very severe. He had in fact been hiding for two days in a cellar when his general practitioner found him and sent him into hospital. As a result of his severe infection he developed kidney failure. Although he was very ill he was mentally clear and adamant that he did not want any form of dialysis treatment.

It was of great concern to us because although acute kidney failure is usually totally reversible, the effects of kidney failure are potentially fatal. We were briefly able to persuade him to have peritoneal dialysis, a technique in which dialysis fluid is instilled into the abdomen via a catheter. After 36 hours this treatment was stopped in accordance with his wishes. His family, who had obviously found his personality problems very difficult to handle, supported him in his view that he did not want treatment.

It was extremely frustrating for the doctors to watch this man die because he refused to accept life-saving treatment of his kidney failure. The position had been explained to him in detail and he had made what on the face of it was a considered autonomous decision, which we had to respect, although we did not think it was rational.

## Autonomy of brain-damaged patients

Problems regarding patient autonomy and the right to decision-making are particularly difficult when patients are admitted to intensive care with altered states of consciousness as a result of brain damage which may or may not be reversible. A retired 77-year-old university professor, very distinguished and with a knighthood, had a past history of disease affecting the blood vessels of the brain. While on holiday in France he suffered a massive stroke. He was taken to the local intensive care unit and needed support with mechanical ventilation. He slowly improved over the next two weeks and was transferred to our intensive care unit. When he was admitted it was apparent to us that he could be taken off the ventilator. The question arose as to how to be certain of his ultimate prognosis and how hard to try to save him.

He had previously expressed the wish that he did not want to be an invalid in a vegetative state. A neurologist was called in who suggested that prognosis could not be adequately judged in the presence of a chest infection – in spite of the fact that the man was 77, that there was a clear evidence on his brain scan that his brain was massively damaged, and that he had shown no evidence of intellectual recovery in the first three weeks.

The family felt that the prospect of him leading a damaged life was not an attractive one. They told us that he himself had expressed the wish that nothing extraordinary should be done to keep him alive should he be grossly disabled or in an irreversible coma. After discussions with the family it was decided not to perform a tracheostomy to facilitate his breathing. It was also decided not to treat him with antibiotics because of his own and the family's wishes. However, we were forced to reverse this decision because his sputum developed a resistant type of organism that could have posed a danger to other patients in the unit. The family were distressed by the antibiotics being given, as they felt this might prolong his suffering.

We have little evidence that patients in this state actually suffer, although intensive care procedures may be very distressing for the relatives. A few days later the patient died, illustrating again the difficulties of prognosis and of rights of patients as against medical opinions.

### Autonomy and irrational patients

A final twist in the autonomy debate in relation to what physicians should do occurs when competent patients make irrational decisions and, for example, refuse life-saving treatment. Doctors may find some patients' religious attitudes frustrating. This applies to groups such as Jehovah's Witnesses, whose religious beliefs preclude blood transfusion. There are situations where transfusion may be a matter of life or death. It is very difficult for the medical team to watch a patient die of anaemia because of religious principles. (On the other hand, it may be argued that objections to blood transfusion may have stimulated the development of artificial blood substitutes.)

The problem arises when a Jehovah's Witness develops leukaemia. The mainstay of treatment of leukaemia is with chemotherapy. This invariably causes anaemia. Should chemotherapy be given, in the knowledge that this will result in anaemia – which the patient will not allow to be treated by transfusion? Similar problems may occur with Christian Scientists, who believe that healing is by prayer alone. On the one hand we may decry the fact that the concept of autonomy has grown up as the influence of formal religion has declined, but on the other hand there are religious groups, as illustrated here, whose principles bar their adherence to benefits of modern medicine.

Questions of autonomy are discussed worldwide. In 1990 a court in Israel gave a decision allowing a patient not to be attached to a life-support machine. The patient in question had amyotrophic lateral sclerosis, which is a condition of progressive muscular deterioration which results inevitably in respiratory failure and death. The situation was entirely predictable and the prognosis was clearly known to the patient, who expressed his wish not to have ventilation artificially given to him when he went into respiratory failure. The doctors wanted court approval in order to protect themselves from charges of manslaughter. In this case the court accepted the patient's video-taped request not to be put on a ventilator, made prior to the time when it would become necessary.

It is increasingly accepted that patients have autonomy and the right to refuse treatment regardless of the medical indications and arguments. Doctors have a duty to continue to treat patients regardless of their refusal to accept medical opinions. On the other hand doctors have the right to refuse treatment requests which they know to be valueless. As in other areas of ethical dilemma, it is encumbent on the doctor to be in command of the medical facts and probabilities and to explain the position fully to the patient and or his relatives or surrogates. It is the fully informed patient that can most effectively exercise his autonomy. And although this chapter has dealt with some of the 'negative' aspects of autonomy, notably with patients who refuse, for one reason or another, to accept potentially life-saving treatment, there is another side to it. For the principle of autonomy extends to the right of a patient to request that under no circumstances should treatment be withdrawn.

# 10

## Living Will

The development of increasingly sophisticated life-support technology has raised fears in some people's minds about the possibility of having their lives artificially prolonged against their will if they are incapable of expressing their views. It is against this background that in the United States the concept of 'living will' has grown up. A person, while still capable and competent, makes a formal statement about how they would want to be treated were this no longer the case. In this living will the person directs his physician and other care providers, including his family and any surrogate designated by the patient or appointed by a court, to carry out the wishes set out in the document. Such a will is now legally binding in many states of the union.

The key part of such a living will states:

> If I become unable, by reason of physical or mental incapacity, to make decisions about my medical care, let this document provide the guidance and authority to make any and all such decisions. If I am permanently unconscious or there is no reasonable expectation of my recovery from a seriously incapacitating or lethal illness or condition, I do not wish to be kept alive by artificial means. I request that

I be given all care necessary to keep me comfortable
and free of pain, even if pain-relieving medications
may hasten my death, and I direct that no
life-sustaining treatment be provided, except as I or
my surrogate specifically authorize.

This statement is taken directly from the living will form
distributed by an organization called Concern for Dying,
based in New York City.

One of the problems of such documents is that the terms
used may be open to varying interpretation. The provisions
of the will assume that the physicians involved will have a
degree of certainty about prognosis which is not always
justified, and the definition of what constitutes life-
sustaining treatment is also variable. On the other hand,
the living will has provision for people to be specific about
what treatments they do *not* want, including cardiopulmonary resuscitation (CPR), artificial or invasive measures for
providing nutrition and hydration, kidney dialysis, mechanical or artificial respiration, blood transfusion, surgery (such as amputation) and antibiotics.

Although the concept of living will has no binding
status in Britain, a comparable situation arose in the case of
the distinguished academic sent home from France with a
massive stroke (see page 86). Although this patient did not
write a formal living will, he had given clear instructions
that he did not want his life prolonged if he was permanently intellectually disabled. It caused the family some distress when antibiotics were prescribed because he had
developed an infection with an organism which posed a
threat to other patients in the unit. We were, of course,
prepared to concur with the patient's known wishes, but
clearly we could not put our other patients at risk by so
doing. It is also often difficult to be certain that recovery is
impossible. It is argued that at the time when a severe
illness occurs the patient's wishes might well differ from
the decisions set out in the living will.

Although I have reservations about the living will concept, there are situations in intensive care practice when it is vital to know the patient's wishes at a time when he is unable to express them – as was the case in a man admitted as an emergency with a respiratory arrest from severe pneumonia. We later discovered he was known to have AIDS with associated blindness. He had given a prior written witnessed statement that he did not want further life support. Unfortunately this fact was discovered only after he was already ventilated in intensive care.

Living wills should not become a substitute for sympathetic communication between doctors, nurses, patients, and relatives. Such wills will never cover all the eventualities, and their legal status in Britain may take time to become established. A living will might best be seen as an advisory device and need not necessarily become a legal weapon. In 1992 the BMA expressed strong but qualified support for the concept of the living will. It clearly makes sense to know the patient's wishes and to act on them if at all possible.

A very distressing case where the provision of a living will was carried out occurred recently in the United States. A distinguished retired American general and diplomat had a heart attack at the age of 85 while travelling on business in Russia. He was flown back to his home town. It is almost a routine in the United States to perform angiography, X-ray of the arteries of the heart, on all heart-attack victims. It was done in this case, in spite of the fact that heart surgery is not a routine practice on a patient of his years. No doubt he gave consent to the angiogram, but I wonder whether the risks in his age group were properly explained to him. It is unlikely that coronary angiography would be proposed routinely for a fit 85-year-old in the NHS; on the other hand, one of the charges against British medicine is that it excludes many patients, such as the elderly, from modern treatment.

This man was known to have signed a living will stating

that he did not want extraordinary medical treatment to be given if he was in a vegetative state. Unfortunately, he suffered a stroke as a result of the angiogram or shortly after it. He was half paralysed, but extremely distressed and angry. Although he could not speak, he was thought to be capable of making decisions, and the treatment process was discussed with him. He declined nutritional and other support, was given sedatives and pain-relieving drugs and died a week later.

The provisions of the living will and indeed the patient's wishes had been scrupulously followed. I found this case distressing not so much because of the living will, although the man's obvious anguish makes me wonder whether he regretted making this provision, but chiefly because I felt it was a mistake for the angiogram to have been done. Sometimes a series of investigations are carried out without proper consideration of the individual patient, particularly in the United States, where there is fear of accusation of negligence, and subsequent litigation, if they are not done.

It has been suggested in the United States that it should be mandatory for patients to give directives, on admission to hospital, about life support and other heroic measures. There are several problems about making compulsory such directives as the living will. First, many patients would not be in a fit state to give such directives themselves or have suitable surrogates available to do this – and immediate treatment may be of the essence. Further, making such directives compulsory might result in futile and un-necessary procedures being done on those patients whose wishes are not clear.

In Western societies death is more likely to occur in hospital or some other health-care institution than in the home. The idea of the living will is to allow the patient some control over his final destiny in an impersonal institution. As with many well-meaning pieces of legislation, it is possible, owing to inevitable ambiguities in wording and terminology, allied with fear of litigation, that the living will

might paradoxically lead to more rather than less prolonged and futile life-supporting treatments.

The development of the living will, however, serves to
underline the need for intensivists to be sensitive to the
patient's wishes and to convince the public that they are
first and foremost caring physicians rather than highly
qualified technicians concerned only with pathophysio-
logical research.

A further disadvantage to the living will is that it does
not allow the patient to change his mind. There may be a
difference in attitudes when making a theoretical plan of
one's terminal care whilst one is well, with one's wishes
when faced with the reality of critical illness. Clearly, if the
provisions of a living will are carried out they cannot be
reversed.

# 11

# Euthanasia

The question of euthanasia – mercy killing – bears on the work of the ICU in much the same way as does the idea of the living will: it reflects the fear among many people that the raison d'être of the proliferating technology at the disposal of intensivists is simply to prolong the process of dying. In the United States supporters of euthanasia have used the image of a dying man hooked up to a life support machine accompanied by relentless sucking of the respirator.

In 1989 a working party of the British Medical Association reviewed the association's guidance on euthanasia. Euthanasia was defined as active intervention to terminate life. They stated that there is a distinction between an active intervention by a doctor to terminate life and a decision not to prolong life (a non-treatment decision). They have unequivocally declared euthanasia to be illegal.

Many deaths in the United States are thought to be planned by patients conniving with their families and physicians. A *New York Times* poll found that 53 per cent believed that doctors should be allowed to assist a severely ill patient to take his or her own life. There is a widespread fear that people will have their lives and suffering prolonged by medical technology. It has been suggested that the medical profession's repeated and firm rejection of assisted suicide is self-serving and blind to the expressed needs of patients. The public appears to be losing faith in doctors at least partly because of our allegedly paternalistic insistence on preserving life at any and all cost, regardless of its quality.

Assisting death may be defined as an act by a doctor with the deliberate intention of hastening the death of a patient with a terminal illness. This raises numerous problems: pressure from unscrupulous relatives, the prevention of improvement in terminal care, the erosion of the trust in doctors. Perhaps confidence in the medical progression is eroded by the fear of technology, too, with its capability to delay death. I think there is public anxiety that this kind of meaningless extension of so-called life is practised in intensive care.

The question of euthanasia in the United States was brought up again in 1990 in the case of Dr Jack Kevorkian and his 'suicide machine' with which Mrs Janet Adkins, an active supporter of euthanasia, took her own life. Mrs Adkins had Alzheimer's disease and knew that she was deteriorating. It was stated that she faced inexorable and devastating loss of the cognitive ability and independence which gave her life its meaning and that she made a rational decision to terminate her own life. Dr Kevorkian assisted her with his suicide machine, a device that enabled Mrs Adkins to self-administer a tranquillizing drug, which in turn triggered the administration of a lethal substance.

## Dutch guidelines

In the Netherlands euthanasia policies have been well worked out. The Dutch guidelines for euthanasia list four qualifying conditions: 1) Explicit repeated request for euthanasia; 2) Very severe physical or mental suffering, with no prospect of relief; 3) An informed, free and consistent decision for lack of other treatment options, all others having been tried or refused; 4) Consultation by the physician with another physician who is not actively involved in treating this patient, and their decision must be unanimous.

Proponents of euthanasia assume that illness causes unbearable suffering, but there are techniques to control pain in almost all situations – sometimes, however, at the price of shortening the patient's life. The second assumption in the proposals for euthanasia in Holland is that the patient has a right to control the treatment. It is generally accepted that patients have a right to refuse such life-sustaining treatment as intensive care.

The concern expressed in a critique of the Dutch proposals is that legalizing voluntary euthanasia may lead to a danger of involuntary euthanasia, secret euthanasia, encouraged euthanasia, surrogate and discriminatory euthanasia, which could become another tool to discriminate against poor and disenfranchised minorities. In an era of ethical relativism euthanasia is a danger because it subverts the physician's role as a healer. The bond of trust between doctor and patient is rooted in the assumption that the doctor's first duty is to preserve life – which is incompatible with any involvement with euthanasia. Since the time of Hippocrates there has been a fundamental prohibition of euthanasia which lies at the root of the inherent trust between patient and doctor.

In spite of the longstanding ban on euthanasia, it is interesting to note that Lord Dawson of Penn, who, as is known, intentionally ended the life of King George V in 1936, was opposed to the legislation of active voluntary euthanasia on the grounds that good doctors did it anyway in suitable cases and that it was better to keep the law out of the doctor/patient relationship as far as possible. No eminent physician would admit to this today.

Another worrying aspect is that a patient's right to die by euthanasia might become a *duty* to die, which would have fearsome implications as it might lead from compassionate mercy killing to the abyss of genocide.

It may be argued that the difference between withholding or withdrawing treatment and euthanasia is merely one of degree, and there have been attempts to label these manoeuvres as passive euthanasia. I do not think this is fair: euthanasia implies an active intent to end life, which is very different from withdrawing or withholding ineffective treatment.

Doctors should examine the needs and values of patients in a context that recognizes the limits of modern medicine and the inevitability of death. R.G. Twycross, a physician involved in palliative medicine/hospice care, wrote that he was 'not in favour of "meddlesome" or "mindless" medical intervention at the end of life ... and that with the onset of progressive senile decrepitude the burden of living becomes increasingly demanding for many old people.' It then might be reasonable to 'give death a chance' – by not prescribing, for example, an antibiotic if an infection arose in a patient who was terminally ill or in an advanced state of senility. He did not support euthanasia – doctors actively killing patients.*

Recent cases in the United States have established precedents at least in that country that, where there is no hope of recovery, nutrition and hydration are treatments which can be withdrawn in certain special circumstances with the patient's consent. There have been cases where courts have condoned the removal of life-sustaining treatment in non-vegetative patients with severe and permanent mental impairment who had a life expectancy of one year or less; but obviously it is difficult to be certain on this latter point. It has been suggested that patients with Alzheimer's disease are reduced to the level of the simplest mammals. Once again this area is an ethical minefield. Doctors should not despatch patients for the

---

* Twycross, R.G., 'Assisted Death: a Reply', *Lancet* (1990), ii, 796-8.

convenience of others, such as members of the family. It is also possible that today's hopeless invalid with Alzheimer's might be cured by tomorrow's medical advances.

There have been debates as to which treatments it should be permissible to stop in patients who are in a persistent vegetative state but are not terminally ill. What is critical in the discussion of persistent vegetative state is the destruction of the capacity for consciousness, hence the loss of 'personality', one of the essentials of personhood. It is argued that for people in a persistent vegetative state, life expectancy is not an important criterion in determining whether life-sustaining treatment may be withdrawn since there are no benefits from their continued physical existence. Is it morally pointless to continue feeding such a patient – or morally abhorrent to stop? The question is fraught with ethical problems.

### Intent v. consequence

The law stresses intent rather than consequences; the distinction in question is between intentional acts and their incidental (if predictable) effects. For instance, it might be reasonable to give a patient suffering intolerable pain large doses of morphine to relieve the pain, although the consequence may be that the patient's end may be hastened because of depression of his ability to breathe.

These horrendous questions do not often arise for intensive care staff because usually it is possible to transfer the patients in these states away from the unit. Nevertheless, it is sobering to think that a byproduct of intensive care activity is the production of such individuals in persistent vegetative state, the living undead.

There are a number of strands to the euthanasia debate. It is generally accepted that patients have a right to refuse treatment and to make decisions about their life. It is further suggested that if the patient feels his life is not worth living by reason of severe, relentless pain or other forms of unrelieved distress, he should have the right to end his life. It is accepted that the relief of suffering is the cardinal duty of the doctor; therefore why not assist death?*

The question of euthanasia comes up in various guises. Is there a case for continuing life-prolonging treatment in states of prolonged coma, severe incapacity or unrelievable pain? Further, is one morally bound to continue life-prolonging treatment, or if no such treatment is being given, whether and in what circumstances is it ethical to hasten the deaths of such people by administering narcotic drugs? When may a doctor assist death?

In 1992 a hotly-debated case of euthanasia came before the courts. Dr Nigel Cox administered a lethal injection of Potassium Chloride to a patient suffering intractable pain which he could not relieve. He was found guilty of attempted murder and given a twelve month suspended sentence. The General Medical Council found him guilty of serious profesional misconduct, but did not erase his name from the Medical Register as he had acted in good faith and his purpose was to relieve her intolerable suffering by expiditing her death.

A concern about euthanasia is that it may lead to the temptation to move from voluntary assisted death to involuntary assisted death, especially at times of limited resources. Although a doctor must respect a patient's rights, patients do not have the right to demand treatment which the doctor cannot provide with a clear conscience. Euthanasia is just such a 'treatment'.

Ludovic Kennedy, a well known proponent of euthanasia, suggested that 75 per cent of British voters want to see voluntary euthanasia liberalized because medicine can now prolong the process of dying with

* 'Assisted Death: Institute of Medical Ethics Working Party', *Lancet* (1990), ii, 610-13.

diminished quality of life.* Voluntary euthanasia is relevant to the tragic minority of patients whose pain cannot be adequately controlled and who consider their quality of life so low that they prefer to be dead.

Secular moralists suggest that human beings have a right to make such choices for themselves. Most religions, however, would disagree on the grounds that life is sacred and not for man to discard at will – which may prohibit the withholding or withdrawal of treatment by a doctor.

In my view the proper response to demands for euthanasia is to improve medical treatment so as to minimize those requests by improving pain relief and control – adequate techniques for controlling and relieving pain are available but may not always be applied. Better communication with patients and adequate psychiatric help may help to relieve mental anguish and depression. Thorough explanation of the purpose and need for intensive care may help reduce the fear of inappropriate and over-prolonged life support.

This leaves those patients in a persistent vegetative state in whom relatives may request euthanasia. In such cases, passive euthanasia does occur in the UK. This would seem to be an area of public concern and possible legislation, as illustrated by the case of Tony Bland, in a persistent vegetative state for years after the 1989 Hillsborough football disaster.

---

* Kennedy, L., *Euthanasia, the Good Death*, Chatto Counterblasts No. 13 (1990).

# 12

# Intrinsic Hazards of Intensive Care

All forms of treatment in medicine have adverse incidental effects, and when prescribing a drug or advocating a procedure the doctor has to weigh in his mind the possible benefit against the risks involved to the patient. Intensive care is no exception. The untoward effects which occur can be divided into technical problems, errors of judgement and problems arising because of lack of knowledge, and possible adverse psychological effects on the patient and/or his family. It should be borne in mind, however, that patients are admitted to intensive care in a critical state and there is great pressure to try to get on and do something to help the patient, who may in any case be less resilient to these effects because of his underlying serious disease or injury. An ethical dilemma presented by these effects to the doctor is the question of how to react to the problem, and doctors are often accused of trying to hide this kind of unfortunate occurrence.

Sometimes errors occur owing to overwork of the staff of the unit, and sometimes because of a rigid application of a preset treatment protocol – inappropriate use of the easy to follow step-by-step plans of patient management which may pay no attention to the individual patient and his differences from the mean.

In the intensive care unit the patient often has long plastic tubes put into his large veins to measure the pressure in his heart and circulation and also to provide him with feeding. These plastic tubes are occasionally faulty; they can sometimes break and float away in the circulation, and the already sick patient will then have to face the hazards of the search for the tube. A very common complication after the insertion of these lines is the development of infection. This will often infect the bloodstream, causing blood poisoning and so further adding to the problems of the gravely ill patient. If this cause of septicaemia is not corrected and treated promptly, the patient may die.

A clinical challenge is to recognize this possibility of line-related infections. We make it a practice in our unit to insist that these long lines are changed at least once a week. Occasionally, when these lines are opened or drugs administered, air can enter the circulation, and this can cause further strain on the working of the heart. Another technical complication of insertion of these central lines is that the lung is punctured and air leaks into the space between the lung and the chest wall. Air can also sometimes enter the tissues of the chest wall, causing them to swell up and become crackly to the touch; this is called surgical emphysema. Many of our patients require treatment with artificial ventilation. But mechanical ventilation itself may affect the lungs' defence mechanisms and predispose the patient to further infection.

A man of 65 came into hospital with a chest illness that proved very difficult to diagnose. His condition worsened on the ward and after nine days he collapsed and required treatment with a ventilator in the intensive care unit. To get adequate oxygen carriage into his blood, increasingly high concentrations of oxygen were required. Oxygen itself can be toxic, and as a result of the high-pressure ventilation he was given, one of the small air channels burst, with a resulting release of air into the tissues (surgical emphysema) causing him to swell up grotesquely. Application of a technical innovation came to our rescue: if it is possible to oxygenate somebody with a rapid-frequency, low-pressure ventilator, the escaped gases can be reabsorbed. We were encouraged to continue by the fact that the patient remained more or less conscious in spite of the fact that his lungs were functioning very poorly and his blood gases were appalling. However, after three weeks on the ventilator he died. It was unfortunate that he had this surgical emphysema, but it is very doubtful whether this actually played any part in his death, which could be looked upon as the end result of a chronic disease. Nevertheless when untoward complications of treatment occur, members of the intensive care team feel guilty, even if that is an irrational response. This underlines the fact that even well-planned and considered and skilful invasive procedures may cause the patient harm as well as good.

### Mishap

There are many examples of accidental mishaps in intensive care. For instance, tubes inserted to measure pressure in the heart or great veins may arrive in the liver. This is usually harmless, though it renders the measurements valueless. It is vital to X-ray the tubes after insertion to confirm their location. Catheters on occasion pass through the heart wall, usually without any ill effects. Sometimes, even simple procedures such as drawing blood from veins can result in infection that may be difficult to detect in the very ill, the very old or the very young.

Many powerful drugs are administered in intensive care, often through pumps. Occasionally these may fail, administering either too much or too little of the necessary drug. Problems with drug administration may arise for a variety of different reasons, sometimes because of a lack of common sense.

It is recognized that the drug Diazepam is of great benefit to patients with epilepsy. A man presented to casualty having epileptic fits and he was treated with Diazepam intravenously. However, his fits continued and the Diazepam injections were repeated until he had 30mg, which is excessive, especially given intravenously quickly. This precipitated a respiratory arrest, necessitating his admission to intensive care, a situation that was almost certainly avoidable had more sense been used in the administration of this drug.

Patients in intensive care frequently have life-threatening infections. Gentamicin is one of the major antibiotics used. Like all drugs it has significant side effects, the two principal ones being the precipitation of acute kidney failure (which is usually reversible) and damage to the auditory nerve (often resulting in permanent impairment of hearing and balance). A patient went deaf after his life-threatening infection of the heart was cured in intensive care with gentamicin. He sued for medical negligence. These gentamicin-induced side effects are preventable if the levels of the antibiotics are monitored frequently and not allowed to get into the toxic range by adjusting the drug dose. However, it is vital that sufficient antibiotic is given to control the infection.

Sometimes when a number of different drugs are given together to the patient, the wrong dose may be increased, again with serious effects. There may also be undesirable interactions between the drugs. Because of the ever-present problem arising from drug administration, a pharmacist takes part in our daily major ward round in intensive care.

Fluids given for artificial nutrition through a vein may also arrive in the wrong place, such as the peritoneal cavity, causing further medical problems. There are concerns that some components of these parenteral nutrition solutions in themselves may give rise to side effects.

Continuous attention to detail in the intensive care unit is mandatory. The type of errors that can occur may be due to the immense pressure of work, which causes overtiredness among the medical and nursing staff, especially if hours are excessively long. Intensive care staff are almost invariably extremely conscientious, and are usually very distressed if errors occur. Sometimes the staff are too busy looking at the charts and recordings and computer printouts, or too intent on following the treatment plan, to examine the patient with sufficient care. As in other areas of medical practice, the importance of clinical examination of the patient cannot be stressed too much.

Sometimes things go wrong even when the right things are done. For instance, a man in his 50s with high blood pressure arrived at the hospital with a severe attack of chest pain, characteristic of a myocardial infarction (limited heart muscle death due to coronary artery blockage). There were a few odd features, such as the fact that the pain spread into his back and down the abdomen. The possibility of dissecting aortic aneurysm, a tear in the wall of the aorta (the body's major artery) was considered but appropriate tests, namely a chest X-ray and an echocardiogram, failed to show it. The patient was treated with streptokinase, a drug used to dissolve clots. Shortly afterwards his condition rapidly deteriorated, and he died in spite of prolonged and energetic attempts at resuscitation.

At post-mortem he was indeed shown to have the suspected damage to the aorta. The only way this could have been discovered was by doing a CT scan, and even then it could have been missed. It was distressing to realize that the cause of the trouble had been considered but had not been possible to prove because of the misleading information we had from the tests. However, the site of the damage – at the place where the coronary arteries begin – would have made attempts at repair very difficult, and almost certainly would still have resulted in his death. In fact, the aneurysm had caused the coronary blockage. The worry was that the streptokinase given to treat the blockage may have made the dissection worse.

We have seen other instances where administration of these clot-dissolving agents has resulted in massive internal bleeding, causing the patients distress. But there is strong evidence that they help reduce deaths from heart attacks, so they continue to be used. In fact, the first patient to receive streptokinase in our hospital was a man in his 40s admitted with a heart attack under my care. The fact that he was an American lawyer made us feel that we had to be doubly careful to ensure he had optimal treatment in case we were sued. With streptokinase treatment, the signs of myocardial infarction reversed. Unfortunately, he had had an intramuscular injection in his thigh, where he developed a large haematoma (blood clot) swelling, but he recovered and did not sue us for negligence.

Mrs B.C. is a 53-year-old lady who has survived an epic struggle in intensive care following a series of misfortunes. She had a variety of symptoms in various parts of the body. She presented to another hospital with persisting neck pain. Eventually a myelogram (an X-ray via a needle into the back) was done to look for evidence of pressure on the spinal cord. Unfortunately, this was associated with an infection. This infection, occurring within the closed confines of the spinal canal, resulted in pressure on the motor nerve tracts so that she was unable to move her legs or, for a period, her arms. She required a neurosurgical operation to relieve the pressure. As she was convalescing from the neurosurgery she suffered massive internal bleeding, which required over 100 units of blood to be transfused. Eventually, it was felt that the only way her life could be saved was by removing the offending areas causing the bleeding, so her entire colon and some of the small bowel was removed.

The result of this gross loss of her intestine is that she has malabsorption of food and consequently is now extremely wasted, though she has survived. She required intensive care treatment for a month during the period of blood replacement, followed by intermittent positive-pressure mechanical ventilation for a few weeks. She slowly recovered. Undoubtedly intensive care management played a part in this recovery, though she is left with a very severe disability. It could well be argued that all her problems stemmed from the unfortunate myelogram, which in itself was done from the best of motives. Her case is an example of intensive care saving the day after a medical accident.

Technology is continually making possible new treatments. As a result of this, of course, the life expectancy of patients continues to rise in many ways. Death has come to be regarded more as a failure of the medical profession than as a natural event. A case in point is the treatment of some forms of cancer of the lung, in which the main airways are unblocked by the use of the laser. This can result in many extra months of reasonable life.

A 64-year-old man suffering with a suffocating condition, with inoperable lung cancer blocking his upper airways, was treated with the laser, and following this he had a torrential haemorrhage. We were able to support him for one day in the intensive care unit before he died. The medical profession feels a strong duty to support people, particularly when the acute deterioration is caused by an undesired side effect of the treatment. Whether this is a logical use of resources in patients who have advanced cancer is debatable. But what other option is there?

A further twist to the problems of prolonged intensive care treatment is that rehabilitation may be difficult. We have seen a particular form of weakness, caused by damage to the nerves serving the limbs, which reverses only very slowly with time and exercise. This has occurred in patients who were ventilated and paralysed for many weeks. Its cause is not yet clear.

### Legal problems

This raises the question of the doctor's actions when one of these untoward medical accidents occurs. There is a fear that when the patients or their next-of-kin get to know the facts they may sue the doctors. This may seem harsh when it is remembered that the accident was quite unintentional and occurred, as illustrated in some of the cases above, in the course of an heroic attempt to drag the patient back from imminent doom. But the expectations of patients and, more particularly, their families are continually rising – partly, no doubt, inspired by steady streams of news in the popular press about medical breakthroughs. And this at a time, paradoxically, when there is increasing concern about funding for health care. I think the right course of action when one of these accidents occurs is not to hide it from the family; this will only increase anger and the sense of grievance. The facts should be presented in full, explaining the course of action, why and how certain things were done and why they went wrong. This kind of good communication may prevent a great deal of grief all round. In my experience, when an action is brought for medical negligence, it is often inspired by a failure to communicate with the patient or the family rather than by the consequences of the error.

### Mental disturbance

It has been estimated that over a third of patients admitted to an ICU develop a mental disturbance. This has a variety of features including delirium, anxiety, delusions, hallucinations, restlessness and disorientation. Contributing factors involved in its development include restraint, immobility, drug effects, discomfort, anxiety, sensory deprivation and sensory overload. Whether this last is the result of the illness or the treatment is not clear. There are also significant effects on the emotional state of relatives and friends in the ICU setting.

The fact that untoward accidents and side effects are almost inevitable in intensive care underlines the limitations of our efforts and the stress under which the staff operate. Constant vigilance is necessary. We monitor our performance, with regular audit meetings to assess the results of our treatment and to correct any problems. As far as faulty equipment is concerned, the Ministry of Health and the National Heath Service issues co-called hazard warnings whenever any fault is reported.

Advances in medical technology are making monitoring and therapeutic equipment simpler and less invasive – and hopefully they will also reduce the number of untoward effects in intensive care units. The very occurrence of medical accidents underlies the need for the fullest consultation and explanation to be undertaken before starting intensive care. This may be difficult to achieve because of the urgent critical nature of the illness bringing the patient to the ICU.

# 13

# Predicting the Results of Intensive Care

Funds are limited in every part of the NHS, and the allocation of resources to intensive care is crucially important. The ICU is at the leading edge of technological advances in medicine. These advances may be significant in saving lives: we can be certain that they will be expensive. The increasing pressure to use severely limited resources to the best effect may lead to a conflict of priorities on ethical grounds. Clearly, if we are to come to an agreed policy on priorities in intensive care, we need accurate data for predicting results. Over the past few years various systems have been developed to provide this kind of data. Until now it has not been possible to apply these predictions to individual patients – they have been used as guidelines for different diagnostic categories.

As we saw in Chapter 4, a survey by the King's Fund suggested that intensive care patients should be classified into those expected to survive; those whose prognosis is uncertain; those in whom death is probable shortly whatever is done; and those in whom death is apparently imminent. The King's Fund panel suggested that intensive care treatment be restricted to patients in the first two categories, who are most likely to benefit. Detailed and reliable statistics are vital for such predictions to be made, especially if the predictions are going to be used to justify excluding patients on the grounds that they would not benefit.

Doctors involved in intensive care are haunted by the possibility of making a mistake, and are rightly reluctant to make the decision to withhold or withdraw intensive care from patients on the grounds that they are not predicted to do well. It is not so difficult, ethically, to scale down treatment if the patient in intensive care does not progress well; and it is easier still to make such a decision if the medical facts are well grounded. Often those working in intensive care have little control over the selection of patients for admission, which may depend more on the overall activities and specialties of the hospital and on relationships between the intensive care staff and other hospital departments.

### Predictive systems

A number of prediction formulas have been developed that use observations made on the patients when they are admitted. These formulas include the Glasgow Coma Score, which consists of serial observations of the conscious state or neurological status of patients; the Therapeutic Intervention Scoring System (TISS); the Simplified Acute Physiology Score (SAPS); and the APACHE II Score. APACHE II, perhaps the best known, is an attempt to measure how sick the patient is and to express this as a number. APACHE stands for Acute Physiology and Chronic Health Evaluation. Its results are derived from a number of markers of the patient's clinical state as well as loading factors for any previous diseases, and its accuracy has been proved in many different units in many different countries. If the system is used on a daily basis it will permit very accurate predictions to be made, and the data may help guide ICUs in selecting whom to admit, how long to treat them, when to discharge them and when to stop treatment. It may also allow us to replace imprecise terms, such as 'terminal state', with accurate probability predictions.

Advances in computer technology may enable us to establish such probabilities on a continuous basis by linking the patient's monitoring systems and laboratory results with previous data, and they would allow rational decisions to be made about competing entitlements to intensive care. Such a system would certainly be preferable to other methods of allocating intensive care, such as first come first served, severity of disease and, in some instances, ability to pay. But no predictive system will remove the ethical dilemma of treatment allocation or decide who should carry out the allocating.

The quality of predictions produced by APACHE or any other system is governed by the computer world aphorism 'garbage in, garbage out'. In other words, it depends on the quality of the data fed into the computer. If it is inaccurate, the prediction will be worthless. There is also a danger that staff may be unduly influenced by computer predictions, which may then become self-fulfilling.

It has been argued that effort would be better devoted to improving intensive care treatment than to worrying about outcome predictions. However, economic constraints are pressing, and it seems undeniable that there is an important need for such probability data – even though at present it must be applied to the individual with extreme caution.

It may seem strange that mortality *increases* with the cost of treatment – until one realizes that most non-survivors will have stayed longer in intensive care and had far more procedures carried out than survivors. Applying inappropriate – that is, predictively unsuccessful – intensive care treatment not only delays the process of dying, adding to a patient's distress, but is a waste of resources.

My own intensive care unit has been taking part in the national APACHE study, which involves taking scores from each patient's first day. We have recently begun to audit our own data, and I was particularly interested in the mortality rate of acute kidney failure, which often reflects multiple organ system failures. First-day APACHE scores in this small group were the same for both survivors and non-survivors. We have not repeated APACHE scores later on, but one would expect those on, say, the third ICU admission day, to correlate better with mortality. Each APACHE score is an attempt to estimate the severity of a patient's illness at that particular moment, so using a single score as an indicator of prediction, ignoring the fact that this score could reflect an improving *or* a worsening illness seems to be unjustified.

### Humanity and predictive policy

There are a number of conditions in which the mortality rate in intensive care is very high. Typical are the life-threatening complications of malignant blood diseases such as leukaemia. Patients suffering from leukaemia commonly receive chemotherapy treatment, which usually triggers a profound fall in their white cell count, and lower resistance to infections such as pneumonia and septicaemia which may be complicated by kidney failure, requiring dialysis. These complications are predictable and the patient's chances of recovery are remote. An intensive care policy effectively determined by predictive systems would require withholding further treatment from this patient. But for the ICU staff the decision to stop treatment is very difficult, especially if the patient happens to be a young child surrounded by his family praying and weeping at the bedside. Can the intensivist remove their hope of a miracle when statistics tell him the chances are remote? The choice is made even more difficult because a decision to withdraw treatment would not necessarily be unethical. There is a need to balance rational predictions with individualized treatment that takes account of the humanity of the patient and his next-of-kin. It may be kinder and more ethical not to admit hopeless cases to ICUs, provided we can be sure of our predictions.

Major abdominal operations on patients aged 80 and over have a very poor prognosis, but no intensivist would assert that such patients should be barred from intensive care on that account alone. Instead, such advanced age should be accepted as another element in the clinical challenge, while bearing in mind that, if rapid improvement does not occur in such patients in intensive care, it may well be pointless to prolong efforts.

In order to predict the outcome of intensive care in individuals, repeated measurements of outcome markers, including APACHE and Glasgow Coma Score, have been made and a system of ongoing outcome prediction devised. In a study of 831 patients carried out along these lines by Chang and colleagues,* 109 patients were correctly predicted to die. The remaining 722 were classified by the computer as of unknown outcome; of these, 181 died and 541 survived. For comparison with this study, experienced intensive care doctors and nurses were asked to predict death. The computer made no incorrect predictions of death, but both the doctors and the nurses proved fallible. The implication of such a prediction of death might justify the transfer of a patient from intensive care to a facility where he could be treated in comfort and with kindness rather than with aggressive investigation.

This system of individual outcome prediction requires greater precision than it can achieve at present. And while

* Chang, R.W.S., 'Outcome Prediction', *Lancet* (1989), ii, 143-6.

even now this type of data may help to improve the admission and discharge policy of ICUs, it is essential that, even in the future, when the predictive systems have been refined, the computer remains a tool of the intensive care unit rather than its master.

# 14

# Neonatal and Paediatric Intensive Care

Since 1960 the development of special ICUs for babies has greatly improved our ability to care for very small premature infants. At one time many people doubted if keeping these very small infants alive served any purpose other than increasing the population of handicapped children. Studies in various parts of the world, however, show that in recent years there has been a progressive fall in mortality largely as a result of neonatal intensive care. At the same time there has been no increase in the percentage of handicapped children surviving. What has happened is that more normal children who started with extremely low birth weights now survive. It should be pointed out that 98 per cent of the handicapped individuals owe their disability to genetic defects, the most common of which is Down's Syndrome (mongolism); there is no evidence that genetically impaired children are more likely to be born prematurely, although many pregnancies of genetically impaired foetuses end very early by natural abortion.

Imaging techniques, such as ultrasound, nuclear magnetic resonance (MRI) and infrared spectroscopy, which are able to detect and measure brain damage, allow us to make better predictions as to the quality of survival in very small infants. Neonatal intensive care is extremely cost effective and has been a great blessing to thousands of people.

Some authorities have suggested that very-low-birth-weight babies – those weighing less than 1500g (3lb) – should always be ventilated immediately they are born to avoid any risk of severe respiratory failure and before the classic indications for ventilatory assistance become apparent. The 'active' approach to management of these premature infants has resulted in a dramatic improvement in survival. Among infants ventilated for the respiratory distress syndrome, mortality declined from 79 per cent in 1965 to 17 per cent in 1983. A survival of 79 per cent of very-low-birth-weight infants has been reported, the decrease in mortality being related to an important decline in disease and other disabilities. In 1981 54 per cent of infants weighing less than 1250g (2½lb) at birth had poor development of the nervous system and low mental status at follow-up, but a more recent report claimed that only 12 per cent of infants born at 23-28 weeks of gestation were severely handicapped.

Some intensivists and others are worried that this policy of active management might lead to some infants undergoing prolonged intensive care, only to die eventually, with heavy financial and emotional burdens for the family and staff. But a review of the timing of most neonatal deaths has confirmed that intensive therapy is not prolonged without good reason. In two series of cases 66 and 56 per cent of deaths respectively occurred within the first 24 hours of life, and a third report found that 50 per cent occurred within the first 48 hours. If the aggressive approach to the treatment of very small infants is to be adopted, and unnecessary suffering and futile measures are to be avoided, we need to have accurate guidelines and prognostic information to indicate when intensive care should cease. This mirrors the situation in adult intensive care. More and better data on the causes of death or severe handicap would allow us to improve the quality of neonatal intensive care and make better allocation of resources.

### Prematurity and congenital abnormalities

Concern has been expressed that babies born at or before 25 weeks of pregnancy stand no better chance of survival now than they did six years ago. Most of these infants will be less than 750g (1½lb) in weight, and for them the prognosis remains very poor. In fact it may be better to direct efforts towards safely prolonging pregnancy beyond 25 weeks to give the infant a better chance of survival. After all, the optimal incubator is the mother's womb.

Neonatal intensive care units also have to face the vexed question of handling the care of babies who are hopelessly malformed and who have no real hope either of survival or of growing into anything remotely like normal adults. It can be argued that the neonatal ICU is not the place for such infants, who need to be cared for with the greatest love and attention in another type of unit. The questions remain as to how much support must be given to such infants, and whether we are absolutely certain of the prognosis.

Often the real dilemma with these children is whether or not one can justifiably withdraw feeding. This is a difficult issue; there are many very emotional and ethical arguments over it, which parallel the discussions on withdrawal of nutrition in adults. Some parents feel duty bound to protect their offspring at all costs, regardless of defects. On the other hand, when parents care for such an infant at home it can have damaging effects on other members of the family.

The British Appeal Court ruled in October 1990 that a

severely handicapped 5-month-old baby should be allowed to die if he fell critically ill. This has given legal validity to a code widely practised by paediatricians under which treatment is withheld from babies who face a demonstrably appalling future – brain-damaged infants likely to be permanently blind, deaf, paralysed and unable to speak or comprehend what is going on around them, though they are able to appreciate pain.

The issue is not a right to impose death, but a right to choose a course of action which will fail to avert death. Use of drugs or surgical procedures to hasten death would never be justified, but deliberate steps need not be taken to prolong a miserable existence. Another aspect of the dilemma is the possibility that the doctors may be weighing the costs of keeping a baby in an incubator for many weeks and so denying use of that machine to other babies who have a better chance of living a good life. The British Medical Association stated that the best care was using medicine to cure people. If you cannot cure, then a balance must be found between lengthening the person's life and using inappropriate technology which may cause harm. The October 1990 court decision legitimizes what has been practised by many British paediatricians for years.

## Paediatric ICUs

In addition to neonatal intensive care units there is a need for paediatric ICUs for bigger children. Those with needs such as bone marrow transplants and surgery require this kind of specialized support. When these young patients are treated in adult intensive care units the staff do not always have the special skills needed for looking after children. Particular skills in the intensive care of both children and the newborn include expertise in such vital areas of treatment as maintaining the airway free of problems, while experience in managing the small tubes and instruments may be needed. Advances in surgery to the newborn also extend the horizon of possible treatments.

The problems of dealing with dying infants and children are in many ways more painful and difficult to handle than similar situations occurring in the elderly, but often the same ethical dilemmas occur. For example, should children with incurable congenital abnormalities be resuscitated? How much and what should the children be told? Is it justifiable in these cases to withdraw nutrition and hydration? These are recurring dilemmas, though fortunately rare. Hopefully, at a time of limited resources, financial priorities for neonatal and paediatric intensive care will be maintained or increased.

The hospital where I work does not have a paediatric ICU, but we do have a well-known neonatal intensive care unit. When a child is admitted to our adult unit the paediatricians play a major role in the patient's management. A number of our nurses and doctors have received specialized paediatric training. We have had numbers of children with severe forms of croup whose upper airways are blocked as a result of an acute infection – a dangerous condition. We have looked after other children with various problems, including an 18-month-old boy with breathing difficulties caused by an undetected chicken bone in his throat, as well as children with asthma and accidental poisoning or following surgery. Although they have all had significant clinical problems, our staff have enjoyed looking after them and fortunately we have not been faced with ethical conflicts or dilemmas in their treatment. To help a child to recover is a source of great satisfaction to all concerned.

## Parental problems

Another dilemma may arise if the parents oppose the application of effective treatment of their children on religious or other grounds. Christian Scientists, for instance, believe that prayer alone can cure disease. Should the doctor respect the parents' wishes and watch the child die? Parents, of course, have the right to decide and give consent to treatment for their children. A particularly sad case occurred in the United States, where Mr and Mrs Twitchell were convicted of involuntary manslaughter because of wanton and reckless disregard for their son's health. As Christian Scientists, they had relied on prayer to cure their 2½-year-old, who died of a treatable bowel obstruction. Parents have a duty to care for children. If parents do not call for medical help for their child when they know him or her to be ill, this is regarded as manslaughter if the child should die.

In the United Kingdom, in certain cases, if the child of Jehovah's Witnesses needs a blood transfusion, the child may be made a ward of court by the doctors and the transfusion given if the parents refuse to sanction it. In fact, in an emergency, doctors may act as they think necessary, but they must be prepared to defend their actions, so a second opinion is desirable. The rights of parents as opposed to the duty of the doctors to care for sick children is an area of debate.

In 44 states of the United States there is legislation exempting parents from criminal liability if their children are harmed, because they choose religious healing over medical care. Conventional medicine, not to mention common sense, would suggest that prayer plus antibiotics is better than prayer alone. People prayed for thousands of years to make smallpox disappear, but this was achieved by modern medicine; and the analogy can be taken much further.

We quite often see infants brought into our unit as a result of parental problems. In a way, social problems are visited from one generation to the next. A case in point was a child of an HIV-positive mother, who had another child in care. She left this child together with two siblings, all under five, while she went out. The 1½-year-old was later found on the concrete below her home, having fallen or been thrown 15 feet from a window. He showed signs of a stroke and required an operation to drain a blood clot from his brain. It is likely that he will survive, though quite possibly with damage to the nervous system, adding further to his disadvantages.

A similar case was that of a young child of 2½ who was left at home by his single-parent mother together with two siblings. There was a fire caused by an unattended chip pan. Two of the siblings died, but the third escaped; he came into hospital with 45 per cent burns, including an inhalation injury. He is making good progress but the psychological damage will be considerable. A further twist to this unfortunate tale is that the child required frequent blood samples for tests and because venipuncture was difficult, the blood was taken from one of the femoral vessels which are much larger in the groin. When he went to the ward following his stay in intensive care, it was noticed that he had a limp and eventually we discovered that he had a large abscess in the region of the psoas (a muscle that flexes the thigh on the abdomen), presumably the result of his venipunctures.

In intensive care we see the most difficult and therefore least typical paediatric cases. We have had to care for infants who have had cardiac arrests from asthma – in one case, the infant was left in a persistent vegetative state. Another one-year-old had spent virtually all his life in the neonatal unit following very premature birth with poorly developed lungs. He required almost continuous ventilatory support. His parents spent the whole year at his bedside. Unfortunately a series of cardiac arrests left him profoundly brain-damaged. His mother frequently expressed concern that we might withdraw treatment from her child because we needed the bed. This did not happen. The child improved sufficiently to breathe on his own, and was sent to the ward.

The body of evidence of the benefits of neonatal intensive care is very impressive. It is important to realize that the overwhelming majority of children treated in intensive care are going to grow into healthy, normal adults. Many of the ethical dilemmas in paediatric and neonatal intensive care are essentially the same as those in adult intensive care, but they seem all the more poignant because of the youth and helplessness of the patient.

# 15

# Transplant Ethics

Of all the developments in modern medicine, perhaps organ transplantation provides the most ethical problems and the most stimulating re-examination of medical principles. Organ transplantation has obliged us to refine the definition of death. Intensive care touches this field in a number of very important areas. Most organs are donated or taken from patients who are brain-dead – that is, have suffered irreversible brain damage. In the pre-transplant era death was defined by cessation of heart and lung function. The classical common law definition of death was 'The cessation of life, the ceasing to exist; defined by physicians as a total stoppage of the circulation of the blood, and a cessation of the animal and vital functions consequent thereupon, such as respiration, pulsation, etc.'*

The concept of brain death has developed over the years. A Harvard University committee defined brain death in 1968 as the irreversible cessation of all function of the brain, including the brain stem. In a commentary on this definition they suggested that responsible medical opinion was ready to adopt new criteria for pronouncing death to have occurred in an individual sustaining

* 'Death', *Black's Law Dictionary* (1968), p. 80.

124

irreversible coma as a result of permanent brain damage –
in other words, to accept the concept that the individual is
dead when his brain is dead, rather than waiting for the
circulation to stop.

In the United Kingdom the diagnosis of brain death is
made by strict clinical criteria, which are met when there is
no evidence of brain-stem function. At least two sets of
tests are carried out at an interval of some hours by a pair
of physicians, one of whom is a consultant. The tests are
those for any activity of the brain stem, such as ability to
breathe or to react to painful stimuli in the area of the head
and neck. There must be no evidence of response of the
pupils to light or touch and no response to pain within the
area of the head. Normally when ice cold water is instilled
into the ears, rapid eye movements occur, and these must
be absent for brain death to be diagnosed. Finally, there
should be no effort made to breathe when the patient is
disconnected from the ventilator. These tests must be
repeated twice by at least two doctors who have no direct
connection with the transplant team. The tests are carried
out in the absence of hypothermia (abnormally low
temperature) and at least 24 hours after any drugs given
which could possibly have depressed the nervous system.

To my knowledge there have been no cases where
brain-death tests, properly carried out in the manner
described, have subsequently been shown to be wrong.
When treatment has continued despite this diagnosis, all
have died within a short period on full support. Special
investigations, such as X-rays, of the blood supply to the
brain or recording of the electrical activity in the brain are
not required in the United Kingdom.

After brain-stem death has been certified it is
permissible to remove the patient from the ventilator; or, if
consent is obtained for using his organs, these organs are
removed while the donor is still maintained on the
ventilator. In fact, it has been recommended that potential
organ donors are managed in intensive care in order to

maintain the organs in optimal condition: it is possible to maintain good blood flow to the donor organs using intensive care techniques even though the donor's brain is dead. The success of transplant procedures depends on the viability and quality of the organs. There was a case of a young woman who during pregnancy suffered a catastrophic cerebral haemorrhage, causing brain death. It was possible for her pregnancy to continue for several weeks and eventually a normal live infant was delivered by caesarian section. At autopsy the clinical diagnosis of brain death in the mother was confirmed by finding that the cranial cavity was empty.

Many organ donors are victims of accidents, and many are young. Provided the families have time to realize that everything possible has been done to save their loved ones, they often find it a consolation that other people may benefit from their personal tragedies.

### Brain-death controversies

There have been worries expressed about the concept of brain death. As presently defined, the criteria are concerned with brain-stem functions. It is not known precisely which part of the brain is responsible for higher thought processes, and the source of concern is that it might be possible for patients to lose their brain-stem function while retaining some higher levels of function such as thought, feeling and communication. I believe this fear is not well founded because one can usually demonstrate absence of blood flow to the brain in people who are brain-dead. It has also been suggested that, when brain-stem death occurs without evidence of damage to the higher levels of the cortex, other tests such as the EEG (which measures electrical activity in the brain) should be performed to ensure absolute, total brain death. Radio-isotope methods could help to remove any shadow of doubt about brain viability. In the United Kingdom, as already mentioned, the diagnosis of brain death is made solely on clinical grounds, without a requirement for EEG, radiology or radioisotope tests.

The brain death criteria described exclude the possibility of recovery and any kind of independent integrated brain function. It has been argued that brain death is a misnomer in that the brain is in a state of irreparable damage when in fact much of it may not be dead. Further, brain death may be a slogan to allow organ donation from irreversibly damaged individuals.

Some societies and religious groups do not accept the concept of brain death, which adds to the difficulty of obtaining donor organs. We recently had a young Chinese girl, a student from the People's Republic of China, who was brain-dead as a result of a brain haemorrhage. This patient's father wished to come from the People's Republic to see her and a delay of a week occurred. She had been certified as brain-dead within 72 hours of admission. We were told by officials of the Chinese embassy that organ donation is not readily accepted in China. The nurses found it very difficult to accept the fact that we were continuing with ventilation and full support while awaiting the father's arrival – an attitude which I can understand because, if we accept the entity of brain death, there would seem to be no good reason to prolong treatment after this has been declared. In fact, although we tried to continue support, if only for diplomatic reasons, the patient died before her father arrived. (We were later told by her friends that the family would not have consented to organ donation.)

There are some relatives who cannot bear the thought of their loved ones being used as organ donors. I recall the case of a young man on his honeymoon whose new wife died while they were eating in a restaurant. He could not contemplate the idea of her body being violated. Fortunately, today many people are prepared to agree to donation. Often relatives mention their willingness to consent to it even before the subject is raised by the doctors, who may have been emotionally involved in a futile effort to save the patient. On the other hand, it has been suggested that organ donation, with its promise of continuing life, may result in delay of proper mourning by the relatives of the donor. The fact that an organ is still alive may make the relatives feel that the loved one is not totally dead. We try to make sure there is no contact between the donor's family and the recipient, as difficulties might readily arise.

There is a postscript on the subject of brain death. In a study of over 1000 patients with clinical criteria of brain death, it was found that somatic or cardiac death occurred in all of them within seven days despite full support, though others are known to have survived longer.

## Donor organ supplies

In many countries, the treatment of kidney failure and irreversible heart and liver failure and now failure of the pancreas and lungs is dependent on the availability of donor organs. Particularly in the case of the heart and liver, it is vital that the donor organs are obtained in optimal condition for the transplant operation to be successful. In the case of the kidney, it is possible to support the recipient by dialysis while the transplanted organ recovers from any injury received in the process of transplantation. If the transplant recipient develops a medical complication he may well need to be treated in intensive care. This is of course routine for heart and liver transplants. Sometimes the ability to do a transplant operation is restricted by the availability of intensive care facilities for the recipient.

With brain-dead patients providing the organs to treat many people suffering from irreversible failure of the heart, lungs, liver and kidneys, there has been great pressure to increase the supply of donor organs. Successful transplantation can result in an almost miraculous transformation of the quality of life of an individual and be very cost effective; it can return the recipient to fitness and productive life instead of prolonged invalidity or worse.

In order to define the situation in the United Kindom, and perhaps also to stimulate the availability of donors, a study of organ donation from intensive care units was carried out.* Brain-stem death was a possible diagnosis in 407 patients, or 14 per cent of the study; in fact, half the patients with brain-stem death became organ donors. Tests for brain-stem death were not performed in 106 cases. Consent for organ donation was given by 70 per cent of those asked.

There seems to be a need to carry out more brain-stem death tests in potential organ donors and also to improve public education to increase the rate of consent. Nowadays it is routine to ask for consent to remove a range of organs for transplantation when a donor becomes available. In half of those donors in the study from whom there was permission for multi-organ donation, only the kidneys were removed. The authors of the study suggested that more organs are lost as a result of transplant team logistics than by failure to seek consent from relatives of brain-dead patients. Those logistical problems included lack of available surgeons to remove the organs.

An ideal organ donor is someone who is fit apart from catastrophic brain injury or disease. The presence of cancer, other than certain rare tumours restricted to the brain, is a contraindication to organ donation, as is active infection; drug addicts are excluded from organ

* Gore, S.M., et al., 'Organ Donation', *British Medical Journal*, (1989), 299, 1193-7.

donation because of their high incidence of HIV infection. Cancer and viral infections, including AIDS and even rabies, have unfortunately been transmitted by transplant-ation. Nonetheless, in these times of shortage of donor organs, attempts have been made to extend the range of suitable donors and re-examine some previously held contraindications to donation. Intensive care staff must be alert to the possibility of brain death and of organ donation. In the United Kingdom there is a network of transplant co-ordinators, who are always on call and available to advise ICU personnel on the procedure to be applied in the case of potential organ donors.

We recently had a tragic case of a young man who presented to our intensive care unit in deep coma resulting from meningitis. He was treated energetically with antibiotics, but after a few days he was brain-dead. Our microbiologists assured us that his infection had been eradicated. After obtaining consent from his family, his kidneys were removed and they have been successfully transplanted to two patients. Only one kidney unit in the United Kingdom was prepared to use these organs because of ungrounded fears of infection. I think this case points a way to increasing the number of potential organ donors by reassessing some of the contraindications to donation. It may be that an audit of brain-dead patients in intensive care units would stimulate the use of more donor organs and call into question why some potential donors are rejected.

Another equally tragic case was the death of a young man of 20 who went out to celebrate his birthday on a hot summer night at a well-known London nightclub. He had a few pints of beer with his friends and was given Ecstasy, a drug which belongs to the amphetamine family. He came to the hospital with a very high fever (44°C) and extremely high blood pressure, and he rapidly developed a cerebral haemorrhage which resulted in brain death. As part of this picture, he developed rhabdomyolysis, a condition of muscle breakdown that releases the protein myoglobin, which causes injury to the kidney. At the time when he was declared brain-dead, tests showed his kidney function was grossly impaired but that the damage was reversible. I pressed the surgeons to consider using his organs for transplanting; acute kidney failure is almost always recoverable provided the cause has been eliminated. His kidneys were used with success.

Because of the need to increase the supply of donor organs, other possibilities have been explored, including the use of organs from people who are dead on arrival at the hospital from trauma or gunshot wounds. As yet the results of such efforts are not clear.

Many patients admitted to hospital with severe brain injury – for instance from massive cerebral haemorrhage – are considered unsuitable for intensive care or mechanical ventilation because this treatment is unlikely to be of value to them; many of these patients will later become brain-dead. It has been suggested that it is reasonable to manage organ donors in intensive care and Feest and others* have developed a protocol to transfer such potential organ donors to the ICU. This arrangement applies only to patients already considered medically suitable as donors, and whose relatives have agreed to donation and to supportive measures to facilitate this. In the study reported by the Feest team, over a period of 19 months 8 patients were identified and 21 organs retrieved. This was effectively twice as many organs as had been secured annually for several preceding years from normal ICU practice in that hospital.

### Ethical objections

Some anaesthetists and nurses are not prepared to ventilate

---

* Feest, T.G., et al., 'Organ Donation', *Lancet* (1990), 335, 1135.

patients with the specific intention of providing donor organs. One reason is their reluctance to embark on a major intervention whose essential objective is to secure healthy donor organs rather than to help the patient recover; another reason is unwillingness to commit professional time and other ICU resources in these circumstances. ICU staff are also concerned that the search for donor organs will merely prolong the patient's process of dying if the full criteria of brain death are not met.

There have been worrying attempts to broaden the definition of brain death in order to increase the number of organs available for transplantation. For instance, a new set of ethical problems has arisen regarding the possibility of using anencephalic infants as organ donors, especially for newborn recipients. Anencephaly is a condition in which an infant is born without proper development of the hemispheres of the brain. These infants usually survive only for a very short time, and the question has been raised as to whether they can be regarded as brain dead from birth on the grounds that they show no evidence of higher brain function. A study was carried out in California where brain death was awaited in 12 anencephalic infants. However, because of other complications occurring, organs could be used from only two of them.* This suggests that this type of donation is not only ethically repugnant because the patients are not brain dead but also that it is impractical.

It was also suggested† that anencephalic infants are uniquely different from other handicapped newborns and could therefore be used as organ donors without meeting the full brain-death criteria. This has renewed the debate as to the nature of brain death. There is a view that the

* Medearis, J.N. and Holmes, L.B., 'Anencephalic Infant Organ Donors', *New England Journal of Medicine* (1989) 321, 391-3.
† Truog, R.D. and Fletcher, J.C., 'Anencephalic Organ Donors', *New England Journal of Medicine* (1989) 321, 388-91.

hallmark of personhood is active capacity for consciousness. Hence, anencephalic infants, who lack the substratum of consciousness, are not 'persons' but belong to a different category. An alternative definition is that the hallmark of life is the functioning of the whole brain, which is lacking in anencephalics, in whom somatic death is uniformly imminent.

This idea is certainly a departure from the established criterion of brain death. If an anencephalic infant is able to breathe on his own, he is by definition not brain-dead, and he may have some reactions to pain. The situation is complicated by the fact that the diagnosis of anencephaly can be confused with other congenital abnormalities, such as microcephaly, where the head is very small, or hydroanencephaly, where again the prognosis is different. To some it is ethically unacceptable that these defective infants be regarded as if they are already dead. There is at least a 10 per cent incidence of other abnormalities occurring in anencephalic infants, making their organs unsuitable for transplantation. Personally I am sure that these attempts to use anencephalic infants as organ donors without the usual criteria of brain death should be condemned.

The concept of removing organs from anencephalic infants opens up nightmarish possibilities. It might next be argued that organs could be removed from other individuals in whom death is imminent, such as prisoners condemned to death or incompetent patients in a terminal state, including babies with organ failure and patients in a persistent vegetative state. For these reasons, most authorities react with horror at the thought of using anencephalic infants as organ donors before they are fully brain-dead.

The demand for donor organs has produced other dubious ideas as to how to increase the supply, including the suggestion that, instead of consent required to take organs for transplantation, the situation be reversed, so that organ donation would be compulsory unless there were clinical contraindications or family objections.

The demand for donor organs has introduced a number of other pressures. In the United States it has been suggested that rewards be given to families who donate organs from their loved ones. Such incentives have included concessions on income tax, inheritance tax and the medical costs of the terminal illness, as well as a widow or widower's pension for the remaining spouse and benefits on health insurance and even funeral expenses. These financial incentives might seem plausible, but they could lead to abuse, either of donor criteria or of the proper care of the dying. In view of the ethical problems which have arisen in relation to the sale of organs from live donors, these financial incentives to the families of dead organ donors are likely to lead to undesirable consequences and pressures on dying patients. Such measures have not been introduced or suggested in the United Kingdom, nor in my view should they be. Money is a very undesirable motive when it comes to organ donation. Progress is needed to prevent organ failure.

### Live donors and others

In the case of kidney transplantation, it is possible for first-degree relatives – siblings, parents and children – to act as donors. The same is true for transplants of organ segments. But kidney, and indeed segmental liver, donation by live related donors is not without risk. There are claims that some donors have died, although no such deaths are known to me or to a number of my colleagues who are active in the field. From large series of live donors it has been shown that major donor complications, such as bleeding, thrombosis or septicaemia, occur rarely; minor complications occur in about 12 per cent of donors.

Long-term life expectancy for live kidney donors is not significantly reduced. A case has been reported where a woman donated a kidney and developed renal failure requiring a transplant herself 22 years later. There are major ethical objections to live donation, as not to harm a patient is considered one of the prime ethical duties of the doctor. Surgical operations should not be harmful in intent. In the case of kidney or liver donations by a live related donor, his physical injury (that is, removal of the organ) is justified by consent, although medical advantages accrue only to the recipient. Clearly, the donor must be made fully aware of any risk, and he or she must agree willingly to accept that risk. There should be no hint of any financial compensation, and it is important to be on guard against psychological or even subtle economic pressures exerted on suitable donors by other members of the family.

Organs may be transplanted from a donor to a recipient if there is no blood group incompatibility – that is, if it is possible to transfuse blood from donor to recipient. There are other methods of matching donor and recipient by matching the white cell tissue-typing characteristics. It is possible that siblings may have identical histocompatibility antigens. It has even been suggested, if there is a family group of potential live donors, that consent be obtained and the donor selected prior to the results of any tissue-typing matching procedure to reduce the amount of pressure. It may be that if there are several possible donors the one with the best match may be the least willing. If there is any doubt on the part of the donor, the patient, or indeed of the doctor, the operation should not take place.

Of much more concern is the situation where kidneys have been donated by persons who are unrelated to the recipient. Organ transplantation between spouses has been generally accepted. I have met a young man who donated a kidney to his uncle and then resented the fact that the uncle refused to support him financially. In the

United Kingdom live organ donation is carefully supervised, especially if it involves anyone other than first-degree relatives.

Unrelated individuals have been paid to donate their organs. This has resulted in undesirable complications, including even blackmail. Unfortunately, there have been occasions when such financial dealings have also involved the transplant medical team. Here, there is none of the altruism which motivates the living related donors.

In many countries the buying and selling of kidneys has been made illegal. It has been argued, however, that forbidding the sale of organs may amount to ethical imperialism. For some people in Third World countries the possibility of selling a kidney may be a realistic way of escape from the direst zones of the poverty trap. The idea of the poor man selling his body for the benefit of the rich man is ethically and morally repugnant and increasingly condemned (though such condemnation is loudest in the more prosperous First World). In desperation, kidney failure patients have travelled to Third World countries to buy their transplants. Unfortunately, the standards of care in these countries are often not of the highest, particularly in those institutions condoning the sale of organs. Cases have been reported of recipients of such organs acquiring hepatitis B and HIV, and there have been many post-operative deaths. A further concern is that if organs such as the kidney, where the donor has another organ to keep him going, are bought and sold, the next step is to extend the practice to unpaired organs such as the heart or liver. In other words, to demand the supreme sacrifice on economic grounds. It has been reported that in China kidneys from executed prisoners have been sold for transplantation. Trade in human organs has to be condemned as utterly repugnant.

There are surgeons who refuse to perform live donor kidney transplants even between first-degree relatives on the grounds that it is not justifiable to remove a normal kidney from a person when kidneys may be obtainable from cadaver donors.

## Transplantation

Organ transplantation has become increasingly successful and is now a realistic treatment for failure of the kidneys, heart, lungs, liver, pancreas and cornea, with work in progress on other organs, such as the intestines and even brain cells. Transplantation of bone marrow is successful in the management of leukaemia and other forms of blood malignancies. Patients are often treated in the intensive care unit in the immediate post-operative period following organ transplantation. It is a mark of progress that intensive care is no longer routinely required for all patients receiving kidney transplants. Transplant recipients must be treated with immunosuppressive drugs to prevent organ rejection and failure. These drugs may compromise the recipient's defences against infection and increase the incidence of malignant tumours. Infection in immuno-compromised patients may be very severe and result in organ system failure requiring intensive care.

Allocation of donated organs for transplantation, like allocation of other scarce medical resources, presents a range of ethical dilemmas in some respects similar to that of allocation of intensive care treatment. In these situations life or death may hang on the doctor's decision. But is he equipped or qualified to make this decision? It has been suggested that doctors have idiosyncratic values, coloured as they are by medical concepts and their commitment to individual patients; and, regarding that commitment, what does the doctor do when he has to choose between two patients, both of whom are under his care?

Transplant surgeons and others have grappled with these problems and various principles have been suggested as to how to allocate the organs. The first considers the question of medical need. Should the organ be given to the most critically ill patient? Or may this be a waste of a scarce donor organ? It has been suggested that second heart or liver transplantation should not be done because the results are so often unsuccessful, and there are so many other potential recipients who have not received one. Should the organ be given so as to achieve the best medical result? This sometimes happens when institutions want to show good results and preferentially choose patients whom they think are most likely to do well, but who perhaps have the least pressing need.

Other medical criteria have been proposed, such as the tissue-type matching Histocompatibility Locus Antigen (HLA), but the correlation of HLA typing and successful results of organ transplantation is still debated, especially in relation to cadaver donors as compared to live donors. It may be that too strict adherence to this criterion may result in an unfair distribution of organs, and that some patients who have unusual tissue HLA types will never get them at all. This may relate to the race of the recipient, and there have been suggestions that minority groups are unfairly treated in transplant programmes. There may also be gender bias; while recent evidence seems to support the view that donors should be matched with recipients for age in order to achieve optimal results, certainly in the field of kidney transplantation.

Other, non-medical factors may bear on the allocation of organs, such as the relationship between the doctor and patient or, in some countries, whether the patient can afford to pay for the transplant operation – not the organ, but the hospitalization and medical and laboratory fees. It is commonplace nowadays to hear of appeals for organ donors for desperate and deserving cases. This may represent a form of queue jumping, and probably should be curbed. Other techniques are sometimes applied by potential recipients to speed up or increase their chances of getting an organ, such as registering with more than one transplant programme, and sometimes even in more than one country.

It has been suggested that the social worth of the recipient should be taken into account in allocating organs, but who is to judge this? A form of judging social worth took place in the early days of kidney replacement therapy when dialysis facilities were scarce and committees were set up to select patients, especially in the USA. Interested parties such as doctors, nurses and social workers, as well as community figures such as clergymen, sat on these committees. This was an invidious system giving rise to a lot of justified ill feeling. The committees were accused of being white, middle class and prejudiced against minorities and the under-privileged.

Other principles of organ allocation which should be considered, and in many places are already used, are criteria such as waiting time for the organ, and sheer chance – random selections among patients who are thought able to benefit. It is of the essence that principles of justice are seen to operate in organ allocation. It is this question of justice in allocation of medical resources that has been predicted to become the dominant issue in medical ethics in the 1990s.

A possible answer to the ethical dilemmas of living and cadaver organ donation and allocation may come with the development of techniques of xenografting – that is, using lower animals as organ donors. The technical problems of carrying this out have not yet been solved. Then a new set of ethical dilemmas would certainly arise, spearheaded no doubt by animal rights groups.

# 16

# Medical Ethics and Religious Belief

There is a wide range of religious attitudes to death. Faith has an important part to play, even in this secular age, in intensive care. It is recognized that the religious beliefs of intensivists may influence their practice. Professor Vincent's review of European intensivists showed that their attitudes were affected by whether or not the intensivist was a believer. All creeds concern themselves with the meaning and purpose of life and address the question of whether it is permissible to decide the time of one's death. Many have strong views against euthanasia. Not only active euthanasia is proscribed: some theologians will not countenance any action which may shorten the patient's life, even if the purpose of the action – giving a powerful narcotic, for instance – is primarily to relieve pain rather than to depress respiration, which is an inevitable side effect. On the other hand, some religions hold that extraordinary care – that is, special measures such as dialysis or mechanical ventilation – is not morally obligatory if it is thought to be medically impossible or futile.

The physician's whole career is spent in fighting disease. The fact that death is always the ultimate victor does not change this; on the contrary, it induces in many physicians an almost Churchillian determination to fight death at all costs and to the bitter end. Each death may come to be seen as a failure. This frequent acquaintance with such failure can demand, psychologically, an even greater clinical objectivity which may raise barriers to conscious spiritual care and concern. There must be a point at which death is accepted. Modern medical technology, which may artificially prolong life in an impersonal way, has been accused of constituting an assault on the dignity of the person.

## The role of the pastor

Patients often have anxieties and guilt feelings regarding death which they and their families need to express – not always easy in the context of intensive care. Physicians have a role in creating an environment which accepts and respects human mortality. G.R. Selby, writing about the spiritual care of the dying patient, notes that the physician is more likely than the pastor to be with the patient at death.* He comments further that often the pastor is not allowed into the room where an old person is being resuscitated. The pastor is the physician of the soul and perhaps should be given a place in intensive care, too.

I think that the pastor or hospital chaplain of the relevant denomination has a very important role to play, not only for the dying patient but also for the grieving relatives. I remember the case of a young man who was dying after a long fight against cancer. The family called for the priest to administer the last rites, while a young intensivist was performing his final cardiac output measurements and manipulations. I remember this intensivist drumming his fingers with impatience on the bed table while the last rites were administered –

* Selby, G.R., 'The Spiritual Care of the Dying Patient', *Ethics and Medicine*, (1989) 5 (3), 38-40.

appallingly arrogant and insensitive behaviour by the intensivist whose whole training, one would assume, had given him a respect for the well-being of the patient. I also recall two parish priests who attended the final hours of a young choir boy who was dying of a sudden over-whelming infection. They were almost enthusiastically encouraging the boy's soul to leave for its place in the world to come. I personally found this disquieting, but it seems to have been of great help to the patient and his family.

## *'Allowing' and 'causing' death*

Theologians are concerned with the moral distinction between purposefully allowing someone to die and intentionally causing their death. They hold life to be sacred, and the question is whether there is an absolute duty to prolong it by any means, or whether this principle may be amended in some circumstances. This is a very important area of theological thought and various religions differ in their view as to how strongly life is regarded as totally sacrosanct. The question of the ethical legality of withholding treatment which may be potentially life-saving is debatable. Some authorities refuse to acknowledge any difference between active killing and withholding potentially life-saving treatment. Then there is the problem of double effect, in which an action can achieve good effect only at the risk of causing incidental but unavoidable harm.* An example might be the giving of morphia to a patient with intractable pain, caused by terminal cancer. The morphia will alleviate the pain, but it may shorten the patient's life by depressing his breathing.

* Oppenheimer, H., 'Handling Life: Does God Forbid?', *Doctors' Decisions*, (1989) ed. G.R. Dunstan and E.A. Shinebourne, Oxford University Press, 205-14.

Giving food, water and nursing care are regarded as ordinary means of prolonging life, and there are precedents today for the removal of such ordinary means of support. Examples of withdrawing extraordinary means of support include not performing an operation, which might in itself be life-threatening, in a hopeless case; or not adding treatment such as dialysis.

The definition of extraordinary methods may vary from case to case, and today's extraordinary may be tomorrow's routine treatment. It has also been suggested that if one form of support, say mechanical ventilation, is withdrawn, and it becomes apparent that the patient will not survive, the further administration of substances to support blood pressure, cardiac output, metabolism or renal funtion is pointless, and all these should be withdrawn. But such actions are difficult to follow in practice. Above all, sensitive reactions to the patient's needs for the relief of pain, communication and care are of the utmost importance. I understand that Catholic and other Christian teaching do not require extraordinary methods of treatment to be applied.

Euthanasia is not accepted by the vast majority of religions. The Pope has declared that, according to Christian teaching, suffering, especially suffering during the last moments of life, has a special place in God's saving plan. The Christian tradition uses the term 'stewardship' in referring to the nature of our responsibility for the limits of our dominion over ourselves.

Appropriate and inappropriate stewardship can be illustrated by action and omission, which may appear as killing and letting die. This does not imply that a decision in favour of killing is permissible in situations where a decision not to maintain life is acceptable. This distinction between acts and omissions enshrines a crucial moral intuition concerning what we can and cannot reasonably expect from each other. We expect doctors to exercise, in difficult situations, that common stewardship for life shared by us all, and taking steps to alter the agreed bounds of that stewardship would have profound effects. The public would be deeply disturbed if doctors were legally allowed to assist death.* Such views underline the need for intensivists, many of whom are non-believers, to respect the views and needs of their patients, which may be very different from their own. Doctors do not need to have religious faith, but must respect religious autonomy. Problems may arise when the patient's religious views dictate that he must decline the doctor's advice.

## Jewish perspectives

Orthodox Judaism regards life as a gift of God and belonging to God. As such, life is of infinite value, and this means every minute of life. From this standpoint, euthanasia of any type is absolutely forbidden – as, of course, is suicide. Stopping active treatment also poses difficulties, although circumstances are recognized where it is permissible not to add further treatment measures, as when, for instance, current medical knowledge regards the situation as totally irreversible.

The paramountcy which Judaism places on the preservation of human life is expressed in the Talmud: 'he who destroys a single life is charged as if he destroyed a whole world and whoever rescues a single life is credited as if he saved a whole world'. God created man as a unique creature of infinite worth, and this endows human life with sanctity. Its corollaries are: (1) no human life is worth more than another, or any number of others, and no individual may be sacrificed for the greater good of the community; (2) a moment of human life, being infinite in value, is as inviolable as any longer period of human life.

For many years, this was generally recognized by

* Callaghan, B., 'Assisted Death', *Lancet*, (1990) 336, 1012-13.

people of various religions or none; however, these values have recently come under attack. For instance, Sir Francis Crick, a Nobel Laureate, was quoted in an editorial in the journal *Nature* as implying that we cannot continue to regard all human life as sacred.* Crick suggested that the status of birth and death be reconsidered; a newborn infant should be examined at two days of age to determine whether or not they are an acceptable member of human society. He suggested that in order to persuade people to accept a continuous readjustment of ethical ideas religion should not be taught to children. It is conceivable that one individual's needs might and should be sacrificed for the greater good of other humans. From a biological point of view, it might be argued that human life has no more sanctity than any other creature's conglomerate of DNA. As Dr Seymour Glick, an Orthodox Jew, put it, 'we cannot deny the existence of God-given standards and still expect ethical norms that retain eternal validity'.†

Rabbi Bleich, Professor of Jewish Law and Philosophy at Yeshiva University, New York City, has summarized the Orthodox Jewish position by pointing out that the proprietor of all human life is God Himself and that man is but a trustee of his life. The concept of sanctity of life supersedes considerations of personal freedom. Were autonomy the paramount value, society would not shrink from sanctioning suicide, mercy killing, even consent to homicide.** Bleich adds that, according to Jewish ethics, casting off the yoke of the law is not an act of freedom but its antithesis.

Judaism bestows a privileged position upon preservation of human life as a moral value. This takes

---

* Editorial, *Nature*, (1968), 220, 429.
† Glick, S., 'Human Life and Medical Ethics', *Intercom* (1971), XII, 5-10.
** Bleich, J.D., 'The Moral Obligation of the Physician', *Doctors' Decisions*, (1989) ed. G.R. Dunstan and E.A. Shinebourne, Oxford University Press, 13-27.

precedence over all other religious considerations, prohibitions and obligations except for murder, idolatry and sexual offences, such as incest and adultery. All other Jewish moral laws are suspended for the purposes of saving life, or the possibility of so doing. The quality of life preserved is not a consideration, nor is its length. Ritual obligations for Jews are suspended so long as there is a possibility that life may be prolonged, even for moments. The Talmud teaches that a physician who declines to make use of his skills, or one who gives up his patient as hopeless, is not a physician. The Torah gives permission to heal; it does not give the physician the right to desist from healing because in his opinion the position is hopeless. Rabbi Bleich points out that to depict any human condition as hopeless is to miss entirely the spiritual dimension of human existence.

These duties to help and heal incumbent on the physician apply to all his patients regardless of their origin and faith. This is in agreement with the principles of non-maleficence, beneficence and justice agreed at the Appleton Consensus. Judaism might question some aspects of the principle of autonomy, in terms of declining treatment in situations which are not terminal. It is interesting that a number of ethicists, both non-Jewish and Jewish, dissented from the Appleton Consensus views on euthanasia and the persistent vegetative state and took a more protective view of the value of life.

A physician's training guarantees neither heightened moral sensitivity nor enhanced acumen. Because a patient's condition is perceived to be hopeless, it does not follow that the remaining life is without meaning. God has decreed that we must love, cherish and preserve life in all its phases and guises until the very onset of death. The Talmud in Kiddushin 82A makes the enigmatic statement that the best of physicians are destined for hell – a daunting prospect for the medical profession. This is explained by mediaeval Jewish commentators as meaning that when a physician falls from his high standards of duty, he deserves severe punishment. The other great fault pointed out by these mediaeval commentators, but still relevant to us today, whatever our belief, is that physicians are prone to excessive pride and to assume that life and death is in their hands and not God's. In spite of these strictures, Jews have been attracted to the medical profession throughout the ages. According to the Jewish religion, doctors are required to tender care in all situations and the physician has a unique responsibility. It follows that he may not involve himself in strike action, especially if basic services are endangered. It also follows that the community has an obligation to see that medical services are available to rich and poor alike. The other point of the Talmudic warning that the best of physicians are destined for hell is that the physician must remember that all healing comes from God.

As a Jewish physician working in intensive care, I try to bear these lofty principles in mind. Unfortunately, it is not always possible to live up to them in their entirety. There are many other pressures in the modern intensive care unit: lack of space, shortfall of resources, views of colleagues, and the often strongly expressed views of patients themselves. It is established in medicine that patients and their families have a right to determine or reject treatment, or at least to express their views strongly, and these views may differ from the doctors'. The principle of patient autonomy may give priority to the patient's view, but equally it may protect the sanctity of life.

Islam also has a system of medical ethics which has been developed and evolved by its theologians in consultation with medical opinion. In Islamic society the individual patient is the collective responsibility of the community. Self-preservation is a necessary and integral aim in jurisprudence and necessitates adoption of all scientific methods of treatment. Necessity permits actions which are normally prohibited – for example, if a patient needs to take a treatment derived from a pig (prohibited in Islam), then medical considerations override ordinary religious principles. Islam regards the faithful as an individual body like blocks in a whole building, hence the obligation of individuals in society to help others.

I have quoted disproportionately from Jewish sources; this is because I am a practising Jew myself and am more familiar with Jewish views. But there is no intention in any way to cast any slight on other religions or on humanistic views.

To summarize, principles of medical ethics apply to all doctors and patients. These principles are broadly accepted by all the monotheistic religions, all of whom share a respect for the value and sanctity of life. Problems have arisen between medical and religious ethical views partly because of the increased ability of medicine to preserve life both in infancy and in old age, which has created new situations such as the individual surviving by means of continued mechanical support. Some of the views about making compromises over the value of life may be ethically very dubious, but the influence of religion to uphold ethical views is generally in decline in the West. It is all the more important that doctors, regardless of their own religious belief, or lack of belief, uphold the highest standards of medical ethics, and are at the very least sensitive to the views of others.

# 17

## Value for Money?

The organization of intensive care has grown up as a matter of convenience. There is no absolute reason why patients must be managed in intensive care units; it just happens that the skills they require at certain phases in their illness are concentrated in such units. One looks for clear-cut evidence of benefit associated with intensive care treatment in the United Kingdom, and the question is not whether ICU treatment cannot save lives, which it certainly can, but whether this is a correct allocation of resources. Could more lives be saved by spending the same amount on preventive measures as is currently spent on intensive care?

As an ICU doctor my duty is to care for my patients rather than worry whether this is the best way of spending the health care budget. There is an increasing and I think correct trend for all the sickest patients in the hospital to come to the ICU, because of the concentration of skills available.

Although there is not a clear relationship between prognosis and duration of stay in ICU, some patients recover after months of struggle, while for others the struggle continues in vain for weeks in the face of increasing complications – but it may be difficult to know, realize or accept that the outlook is hopeless.

One of the charges laid against intensive care is that it not only may prolong the process of dying but that it does so at too great a financial cost. An obese businessman, aged 63, who divided his time between London and the West Indies, was admitted to hospital with a heart problem which required the insertion of a temporary pacemaker wire. This was complicated by staphylococcal septicaemia, a particularly virulent form of blood poisoning, complicated by pneumonia. With such acute stressful illnesses, it is not uncommon for stomach bleeding to occur, and this was indeed the case – in catastrophic form. The patient lost 35 units of blood before bleeding was brought under control with laser treatment. He was already in renal failure as a result of his septicaemia, and then he developed respiratory failure as well.

When he came to our intensive care unit he required treatment with ventilation, dialysis, cardiac support, and aggressive antibiotic therapy to bring the situation under control. In fact it was probably the removal of the pacemaker wire, the source of the infection, which helped turn the corner for this man. As he weighed 100kg, it is not surprising that he developed a pressure sore during this illness. After 28 days, he was able to leave the intensive care unit and a month later he was discharged from hospital.

Does this case represent a cost-effective use of resources? His intensive care costs were of the order of £50,000. His long-term prognosis, because of his heart disease, was problematic. The staff of the intensive care unit regarded his recovery as a great success, but clearly this kind of success can be obtained only at considerable financial cost. Does this represent an effective use of scarce resources? I have no doubt in my own mind that it would have been quite unethical to have acted in any other way.

## Quantifying success and failure

In 1989, a study* was carried out in Finland at a number of intensive care units which covered 14,930 patients. Of these, 9.3 per cent died in the intensive care unit, and there was a hospital mortality of 18.7 per cent; in other words, a further 9.4 per cent of the total group died in hospital although they survived the ICU. After six months 31 per cent of this study group of ICU patients had died. However, at six months, 88 per cent of the survivors lived at home and almost half had full working capacity; 35 per cent did not work but were independent; 7.4 per cent needed some help; and 9.7 per cent required continuous help from other people.

It is well established that non-survivors in intensive care use up more resources than survivors. But it is important that success and failure are not measured merely in financial terms. Clearly there is an important financial impact as, in the Finnish study, at six months 46 per cent of the patients felt fully improved, 47 per cent reported that they were partially improved, while 7 per cent said that they were worse than they had been before intensive care treatment. There was no evidence from the study of an increase in the number of dependent invalids.

Also in 1989 a group from the United States reported that for survivors of intensive care the average total cost was $15,000, with a daily cost of $1,074, whereas for non-survivors the average total cost was $26,000, with a daily cost of $1,600. It seems that in non-survivors, more diagnostic tests and therapeutic procedures are carried out as the doctors vainly struggle to save life. The concern in America is that the sum insurance companies reimburse

---

* Nikki et al., 'Long Term Results of Intensive Care', *Proceedings of 5th World Congress on Intensive and Critical Care Medicine*, 1989, Kyoto.

hospitals is being calculated according to diagnostic-related groups; there is a fixed payment for each of these. Intensive care patients incur severe financial losses for the hospital which are worse with non-survivors. This system may act as a disincentive for intensive care, and there may well be pressure from hospital administrators for ICUs not to persist with dying patients.

The treatment of the patient described in Chapter 5 who spent 90 days in the intensive care unit in a private hospital is estimated to have cost between £250,000 and £500,000, owing mainly to the large number of external experts brought in; but this also illustrates the astronomical cost of prolonged intensive care.

In the current climate, the concept of cost effectiveness is of increasing importance in all health care systems, and there are fears that this may well lead to undesirable, continuing and severe ethical pressures. In order to evaluate the effectiveness of intensive care in the United Kingdom, the King's Fund has recommended that a specific member of staff should be responsible for written guidelines on clinical policy in the intensive care unit. They should also be responsible for ensuring that policies are implemented and data collected and evaluated on the clinical outcome and cost, and they should coordinate the clinical care of the patients.

In the United Kingdom the director of an intensive care unit is a doctor whose administrative responsibility has been solely for the clinical care of the patient. He has had very little control over costs of intensive care, which include budgets for nursing and ancillary staff which are usually separate from the medical staff. With the development of the so-called clinical directorates it is becoming easier for the intensive care unit to be managed and planned at a local grass-roots level; the directorates allow the unit to run its own financial affairs, after negotiating a budget with the hospital administration.

## Cost effectiveness: threat or promise?

Many doctors and nurses are worried that intensive care may lose out in the increasingly severe climate of cost consciousness, as is happening with the current reforms of the NHS. It may be that intensive care will be judged to be too expensive and that many patients will not be referred. It may also happen that referring doctors will wait until other patients are virtually moribund before referring them to ICU. It is both cheaper and far more effective to treat patients at an earlier stage, before organ system failure has become irreversible, but this may not happen if referring doctors are deterred by the high costs of ICU.

There have been attempts to quantify cost benefit with the concept of QALY (Quality Adjusted Life Year). This is an attempt to put a figure on the cost of various procedures relative to the expected benefit in terms of cost per year. Quite how the benefit in terms of restoration of health is measured I am not certain. In this notional concept, the figure of £194 per QALY for a scoliosis operation has been quoted as compared to £592 for a shoulder joint replacement and £1412 for a kidney transplant.* I do not know of a comparable figure for intensive care treatment. I find the whole concept of doubtful value.

The QALY represents an attempt to quantify the problem of arbitrary limitation of health care funds. Quality Adjusted Life Years per unit cost are supposed to distribute resources to obtain the best value for money. This leads to absurd anomalies, one of which is that the value of life is implied to be no more than the absence of suffering. Distribution of resources on the best value for

* Klein, R.F., 'Health Economics', *British Medical Journal* (1989), 299, 275-6.

money principle is inequitable for a given degree of suffering. Those whose illnesses happened to be cheaper to treat would be treated preferentially. I do not know of any real-life health care decision in which the QALY concept has helped.

The QALY would lead to a low priority for old ill patients. It would be grossly unfair, because the best value for money treatment for them would be perceived as turning off the life-support machine. Fortunately, this is still ethically inadmissible. But it seems clear that a pseudo-science of health-care economics is flourishing, and possibly competing indirectly for health-care resources. The time and energy spent on rationing systems might be better spent on pressurizing for an increase in resources. This is not to say that I do not accept the need to have accurate data on ICU costs.

The *per capita* expenditure on health care in the United Kingdom is among the lowest in Europe. Most European countries spend a much higher percentage of the gross national product on health care. The problem is that NHS costs continue to rise for no other reason than that the percentage of the population which is elderly is increasing. These people use more health-care resources, and it has been estimated that their cost to the NHS increases by about 1 per cent per year. If we allow another 0.5 per cent for new and better community needs, NHS expenditure must rise by 2 per cent per year over and above inflation, if it is not to lose further ground.

It is agreed that health resources are not infinite, but can the saving of life be measured in cold financial terms? Society in the end will have to decide on the resources to allocate for this purpose, and how the extent to which it will allow its concern with value for money to override all other considerations. It is vital that the concept of cost effectiveness is not permitted to take over from clinical judgement. On the other hand, it has been argued that resources allotted for expensive treatment beget research which, in its turn, increases the demand for such treatment, and fuels the demand for more resources. There is certainly a place for applying good business management techniques to the running of intensive care. But a necessarily increasing awareness of costs of intensive care must not be allowed to lead to the situation where administrators attempt to dictate a clinical policy based on cost limitation.

I abhor the thought that cost might limit access to treatment of patients whose outlook is poor. Many of us working in intensive care recall the occasional recovery in patients everyone thought were doomed. There are many areas of possible cost saving in the management of intensive care units. In our unit we have undertaken a combined study of cost effectiveness with a leading business school. Rather than limiting access, it might be better to adjust management policy after the patient has been given the chance of a number of days' exposure to intensive care. If there were no improvement, a change of policy would then seem justifiable, including transfer out of the unit. There are some dying patients for whom intensive care is inappropriate.

It has been shown that the development of a new life-saving technique or product – an expensive new drug, for instance – may initially seem to increase costs. But if this new measure is effective, in the longer run the money will be saved by reducing the total hospital stay as well as the number of expensive invasive procedures required; and, of course, it may even improve a patient's prospects for survival.

There is a further twist to the cost effectiveness discussion in the United States. Under health care financing administration rules, liver transplantation programmes must show a one-year survival of at least 77 per cent of patients. This will unquestionably put pressure on the programme directors to accept only patients whose outlook is good and to exclude those patients who are less likely to survive.

Although the concept of cost effectiveness has worrying implications when applied to intensive care, it seems likely that it will be so used. It is recognized that costs have to be defined and controlled in health care, and it is reasonable that we should define the goals or effects which we are trying to achieve with treatment. But it would be intolerable if considerations of cost effectiveness were ever allowed to override clinical and ethical considerations in the work of the ICU.

# 18

## Social Victims

With the current policy of emptying the long-stay psychiatric hospitals, we may see more and more people coming into intensive care who are casualties of doctrinaire policy and are unable to cope and look after themselves. Fortunately, nobody has yet suggested that we should make judgements as to whether such people are worth helping. We know that it is rarely possible to cure people of addictions, at least in the present state of the art. A significant number of patients in my ICU come from the homeless of inner London. Many of these homeless people are former inmates of long-stay psychiatric hospitals; others are young people who have come to seek their fortune in the cruel but enticing city.

Many of the patients who need treatment in my unit have problems caused primarily by their lifestyle or psychological condition. Their severe illnesses may be a cry for help for their more basic problems. One such patient was a middle-aged man separated from his wife because of his alcoholism. He had attempted to return to his wife on a number of occasions, but when he succeeded he had caused her physical harm. His wife-beating resulted in him being sent to gaol. He was brought to us from the gaol in a state of semi-coma.

Among the tests routinely carried out in this situation is

one to measure the acidity of the blood, which has a major effect on many functions at a cellular level. He was found to be in a state of metabolic acidosis. This has a number of causes, including excessive consumption of alcohol. He also showed signs of pancreatitis (inflammation of the pancreas causing severe abdominal pain and damage to other organs). Alcohol abuse is also associated with pancreatitis. During his first admission, the cause of this unusual metabolic state was not discovered, but he seemed to be recovering. But then he tried to escape from the hospital. He was caught by the police and returned to gaol.

He came back to the hospital a few days later in a similar but much worse state of acidosis and coma. Among possible causes of this state is swallowing ethylene glycol, a substance used as anti-freeze in cars. We were able to discover that he had indeed taken ethylene glycol. Questions were raised as to how he had managed to obtain this while in prison. Fortunately, he made a good physical recovery. Whether his psychological problems have been improved or helped by this episode is more debatable.

A 46-year-old man was admitted to the casualty department having had an epileptic fit in the police cells. He had been picked up by the police on suspicion of stealing some sherry. He had a long history of alcoholism and he had lost many jobs. There was a possibility that he had injured himself during a fit.

He had suffered delirium tremens on many occasions. This is a condition where the patient has shaking of his limbs, associated with sweating and frightening hallucinations, usually of an animal nature (green snakes, pink elephants and so on), which occur on the withdrawal of alcohol. He had been an artist of some repute and had had a job teaching art in a polytechnic, but had lost this as a result of his alcoholism, and possibly also because of local cuts in higher education. This further deterioration in his social situation had made his alcoholism worse. He had also been depressed because he had lost his home and also because his counsellor had emigrated, and he now felt that he did not have a close relationship with anyone. Following his admission to the intensive care unit he required mechanical ventilation to assist his breathing. However, his fits persisted, and detailed studies of his nervous system with scanning techniques showed that there was no disease in or around the brain which would be amenable to surgical cure. He was weaned from the ventilator, but remained semi-conscious: at best he was able to breathe, but he remained unable to make any sensible responses. There was no question of withdrawal of treatment as he was breathing unaided. He remained in this twilight state for a few weeks until he died.

Many questions arose, firstly as to how he became injured in the cell. One assumed that the fits were a result of accidental injury compounded by alcoholism, which in itself causes fits. It is disappointing that such people cannot always be saved. On the other hand, one is concerned as to how hard one should try with artificial assistance to save people who seem irretrievably damaged. Should they be given antibiotics when they develop infections? How energetically should they be fed? Medical treatment has a momentum of its own. The root cause of this patient's death relates to his alcoholism and social difficulties.

One must be vigilant against discriminatory and doctrinaire attitudes towards patients who are alcoholic. Many other patients have illnesses induced by their own frailty and bad habits – in particular the thousands of deaths from heart and lung disease caused by smoking – yet the attitude of the medical and nursing profession towards smokers is more tolerant than that towards alcoholics. One of the reasons for this is that many alcoholic patients are unreliable, do not comply with doctor's orders, and are manipulative. Although there are organizations set up to help alcoholics with their problems, it is often difficult to convince them that they *have* a problem, and even more difficult to get them to keep up good resolutions, particularly when their personal difficulties persist unchanged. The question of solving the social problems, which certainly aggravate if they do not actually cause the alcoholic's difficulties, is beyond the scope of this book. But it is imperative that alcoholics are given the full support of intensive care regardless of their problems and behaviour.

My intensive care unit admits drug addicts from time to time. Their admission is usually precipitated by infection. This can be caused by their use of unsterile needles for injecting themselves or when the injection sites become infected, possibly because the drugs are made up with unsterile water. Many drug addicts share needles, and this has unfortunately resulted in a high incidence of infection with hepatitis and sometimes with the AIDS virus, too.

Many addicts come to intensive care in a very bad state of health. Sometimes they have acute bacterial endocarditis. This infection causes the kidneys to fail temporarily, so they may require dialysis, and extensive physical treatment, with drugs and even cardiac surgery, may be needed. These patients are frequently difficult to treat: they manipulate the staff, and their long-term outlook is usually very poor because of the difficulty in curing the addiction and the associated social problems.

We sometimes admit patients who have taken overdoses of drugs in suicide attempts. It is our policy to support their vital functions until they gain a sufficient level of consciousness to benefit from psychiatric consultation. At this point they are usually discharged to the care of the psychiatrists.

From time to time we treat patients suffering from self-inflicted burns as a result of their mental or social problems. In the early stages after a severe burn there is a great loss of body fluids from the burnt surface and the patient requires very careful and frequently adjusted fluid replacement. It is quite common for burn patients to be suffering from the effects of smoke inhalation. This injury can lead to rapid swelling of the air passages, and the patient will then need an artificial airway to be inserted and mechanical ventilation. Prompt recognition of airway problems is vital.

We saw such a burn in a young woman of 24, who had a long history of psychiatric illness. As a result of some traumatic situation, she set herself alight. She was treated in our unit at the same time as the victims of the King's Cross Underground fire disaster in which 31 people lost their lives. The mother of this girl came into the ward and said that she felt like hitting her when she saw her injury and compared it with how the victims of the King's Cross fire disaster had been burnt. It is a problem and a challenge for the staff of the unit to refrain from such value judgements in this kind of situation. It may well be that the daughter's problems originated from a painful relationship with her mother. (As it happens, the majority of the patients burnt in the King's Cross fire disaster did not require intensive care; only four of the most severely burnt people remained in intensive care for more than 24 hours, and only one of these died. However, their long-time outlook, and particularly their psychological adjustment, may be very difficult.)

Another form of self-abuse which may result in the patient needing intensive care is the condition known as anorexia nervosa. Associated with fear of weight gain, its victims often abuse laxatives, diuretics, and on occasions thyroxine. Some associated food fads, for instance eating carrots to excess, can cause biochemical disturbances. As a result of these habits, the balance of salts in the body may become profoundly disturbed. Anorectics may be deficient in substances such as magnesium and potassium, which in turn causes further problems. Such a case was a woman who had been abandoned as a child, and later had an unsuccessful marriage. She arrived at my ICU very ill with abdominal pain, diagnosis of which was obscure. She was in a grossly abnormal nutritional state, complicated by a lack of essential salts. An operation had been carried out to try to find the cause of the pain, but apart from some abscesses, no obvious cause was found. In spite of intensive care treatment with assisted ventilation, antibiotics and parenteral nutrition, she deteriorated and died. The primary cause of her problem had almost certainly been the fact that she was anorectic and abused both purgatives and diuretics.

Although our aim in intensive care is to improve and support the physical condition of our patients, we try to be aware of their psychological needs and give appropriate support. Sometimes patients become depressed as a result of their time in intensive care; sometimes their recovery is complicated by delirium or confusional states, leading to behaviour that tests the sympathy of the ICU staff. But we strive to do our best for all our patients, regardless of their personality difficulties and problems, and try never to be prejudiced against the unfortunate. We guard against the attitude that it may not be worth expending health care resources on someone because he is a chronic alcoholic and his chances of recovery are remote. The trouble is, these people may be discriminated against elsewhere and so do not get to be referred to us at all.

# 19

# Research

It is obvious that there is a need for research into the medical problems seen in intensive care to enable us to understand disease processes more thoroughly and, hopefully, to lead to better methods of treatment. It is essential that most of this type of research is carried out on the patients (animal models in most cases are not adequate to answer the kinds of problem seen in our patients). It is equally important that these studies or experiments be properly supervised and controlled. For this purpose, the research ethics committee has developed.

A research project begins with an idea or hypothesis; previous and background work in the subject area must be reviewed, and there must be a clear purpose to the study, with a defined result or aim. The research proposal must be approved by the ethics committee, and the patients or subjects should give their informed consent to taking part.

In normal medical practice the sole intention of any treatment is to benefit the individual patient, not to gain knowledge of general benefit – though such knowledge may incidentally emerge. In medical research, on the other hand, the primary intention is to advance knowledge, so that patients in general may benefit; though the individual patient may or may not benefit directly. The interests of the individual patient are traded off against the interests of other patients and society in general. Because of the obvious ethical problems, patients, doctors and society need a proper framework for research.

Ethical problems abound in the conduct of research on patients in the intensive care unit. There is no doubt that research is vital if we are to make progress in the care of the critically ill. On the other hand, the critically ill almost by definition are unable to give informed consent to the conduct of research experiments on themselves.

### Ethics committees at work

The incentive for the development of research ethics committees to supervise and control human medical experiments derives from two principal sources. The first was abhorrence of the unethical medical experiments carried out by the Nazis on Jews in concentration camps before and during World War II, and a determination that such practices must never occur again. The second has been the ever-increasing pace and extent of medical research, so that there are many new developments which need critical evaluation.

The research ethics committees have concerned themselves with the question of consent to experimentation and with all the ramifications of problems of research involving patients. In the United Kingdom, the Royal College of Physicians has concerned itself with the workings of ethical committees in medical research involving human subjects.* Ethics committees at local level should be made up of people who could contribute a variety of views, including medical members – hospital

---

* 'Guidelines on the Practice of Ethics Committees', Royal College of Physicians Report (1990).

specialists, general practitioners, and nurses – as well as non-medical workers or scientists. It is recommended that at least two persons, not practising or trained in any medical or biomedical discipline, should sit on the committee. At least one lay member should be independent of the institution or the health authority served by the committee, and both sexes should be represented on the committee. It should be of a manageable size. The committee should have the power to co-opt others when necessary for special problems.

Applications to ethics committees must be made in a formal way; the purpose and duration of the project must be specified and the potential hazards to subjects identified. The manner in which the subject's consent will be obtained is also a necessary part of the ethical committee submission. Any interest, such as profit, personal or departmental, financial or otherwise, relating to the study has to be disclosed. It is required that reviews and progress reports of the research must be submitted regularly to the ethics committee. Many medical journals will not publish research work on human subjects unless it is clear that the work was approved by a research ethics committee.

In considering whether to allow a research project to go forward, particularly one involving critically ill patients in intensive care, the ethics committee must feel that there is a reasonable presumption of benefit to patients – in other words that the project is worthwhile. At the very least the research should increase knowledge of the disease (or whatever) in general even if it cannot benefit the subject patient directly. The likelihood of side effects occurring as a result of research should be low.

### Informed consent

Patients are entitled to choose whether or not they will

participate in research, and obtaining valid, informed, voluntary consent is central to the ethical conduct of clinical investigations. The terms 'valid', 'informed', and 'voluntary' imply that subjects have enough information, in a form that is comprehensible, to enable them to make an autonomous, deliberated judgement whether or not to participate. The obvious impracticability of giving full information has led to the saying, 'There is no such thing as informed consent', a criticism which is most easily rebutted by stressing that all the available information has been given and that the subject fully understands its implications for himself or herself. It is obviously advisable to have written consent for research.

It is recommended that subjects be given an information sheet explaining the nature of the research project in a comprehensible fashion. Any fears of patients that refusal to participate may lead to adverse consequences for themselves must be allayed. They must be assured that refusal to participate will be accepted without question and that they will be treated as if the matter had not arisen.

The idea of informed consent is to protect patients from harm and to respect their autonomy. However, there is little sense in talking about autonomy in the case of incompetent, dependent patients. The guideline should be to ask the question, 'Would the patient want the research procedure to be carried out if he or she were in a position to consent?'

We need to balance the fact that failure to carry out research might harm patients – and indeed might be contrary to the wishes and ideals of patients – against the limitations of informed consent in intensive care. It is necessary for the greatest safeguards to be applied before embarking on research on patients who are unable to give consent. It has even been suggested that such safeguards might include comparable studies of competent patients (this would verify the safety of the experiment) and even attempts to obtain a form of consent from a surrogate panel of patients who approximate to the subjects in demographic and psychosocial characteristics – though the latter is, in my view, impractical in the intensive care setting.

In general, in the case of severely ill or unconscious patients the only research which should be countenanced is that which is concerned directly with the severely ill state and which requires participation of such patients. This is usually the position in intensive care.

The question of who may give consent when the patient himself is unable to do so is complicated. The next of kin is a possible source of consent but sometimes such people cannot be reached. There may be an overriding need to give an experimental drug, for instance; it may be difficult to find a suitable surrogate. According to some authorities relatives, except for parents or guardians, cannot give consent on behalf of the patient; but they can and should be asked to give their informed assent. It has been suggested that a patient's advocate be found. This is often a senior nurse, preferably one not concerned with the clinical management in intensive care. There are situations where, provided the proper consent of an ethical committee has been obtained, it is reasonable to go ahead with the research procedure without consent.

There are obviously areas of enquiry, for instance on the significance of biochemical substances or inflammatory mediators in the process of organ system failure, where such ethical problems do not arise because the research is done on a blood sample. Blood samples in any event are routinely taken at frequent intervals in intensive care, and it is extremely unlikely that taking a very small additional amount more for the research could be in any way harmful to the patient. It is nevertheless desirable to obtain ethical committee approval for all types of research on patients, even in cases where only a small additional amount of blood is required. This is what is termed non-therapeutic research.

In general, the intensive care patient should be told about his participation in research when he has recovered sufficiently to comprehend and he is able to give consent.

Special difficulties arise in the case of research specifically concerned with overwhelming illness or unconsciousness which may occur suddenly and unpredictably. This is a common situation in intensive care. In these emergency situations therapeutic research can be one of two kinds. In the first, it is possible to plan a study because we can predict the type of problem which arises. An example of this are studies of new means of treating overwhelming infection with monoclonal antibodies, which neutralize the effects of the damaging substances released by infection. These experiments should be permitted only with ethical committee approval and assent of the patient's relative or surrogate.

The other type of research may take the form of a desperate new treatment specifically for the patient at hand, who may present the ICU with a wholly new set of problems or who may be failing to respond to all conventional means of treatment. In this situation, where the doctor is clearly trying to save life, he may go ahead and initiate whatever may be necessary or worth trying. An example might be the introduction of a new type of untried artificial lung in a patient who was not responding to any conventional means of support and oxygen was not getting into the bloodstream. In this extreme situation in the United Kingdom neither ethical committee permission nor consent is required provided the doctor is prepared to justify his actions afterwards, when he may well be criticized.

Sometimes there is a conflict between the possible benefits of research and obtaining a consent because, for instance, of shortage of time. It can be argued that failure to carry out research may be unethical, particularly in relation to critically ill patients. On the other hand, patients may sometimes be persuaded by the unscrupulous to consent to irrational or 'quack', unproven treatment. The best intensive care units have integral research programmes on the grounds that it may be harmful to continue outdated and ineffective treatment measures, instead of trying to develop better ones.

Valid intensive care research is often difficult to carry out because of the complexity of the patient's illness and the range of problems it presents. One of the standard methods of clinical research is to conduct a clinical trial, which is a study of two or more evenly matched groups of patients or treatments in which the investigators may not know into which group their patient or treatment has been entered – a blind situation. This is often difficult, because intensive care patients are not uniform, and it is very difficult to obtain a comparable group of patients. Also, many intensive care units see only very small numbers of any particular problem and it may be that reliable research has to be carried out on a multicentre or even multinational basis. Here again problems abound and great care has to be taken in defining the terms of reference for such a trial. The combination of an unconscious patient, unable to give consent, and the complexity of the treatment, means that the potential for abuse during research in the crtically ill is greater than for almost any other group of patients.

It is an accepted principle that if an accident occurs in the course of clinical investigation, the individual patient who is injured is entitled to compensation if negligence on the part of the research worker or his team or a supplier of drugs or equipment can be shown. Since one of the purposes of medical research is to explore the unknown and to discover if there are any unforeseen or unforeseeable consequences of the investigation, accidents may occur, despite the greatest care. The problems of research involving patients have been discussed in a further publication of the Royal College of Physicians.*

* 'Research Involving Patients', Royal College of Physicians Report (1990).

## 20

# Decision-Making:
# Some Success Stories

Intensive care units vary considerably, reflecting differences in populations served and the mix of cases; for this reason it is difficult to make direct comparisons between units. Various means have been devised: one of them, for instance, uses the APACHE score (see page 111), which represents an attempt to quantify severity of illness, to help make comparisons between different conditions and different units. The value of such scoring systems obviously increases if they are used repeatedly. If a patient arrives critically ill, he may have a high APACHE score; if treatment is sucessful by the next day, that score will have fallen considerably. It is far better to rely on several APACHE scores rather than a single one as a guide to prognosis. Collection of such data is work-intensive because of the number of variables and the need to repeat the task daily.

Mortality rates vary in different intensive care units. In an audit of the first five years' work in a new intensive care unit, 1483 consecutive patients admitted to the unit were reviewed. The largest admission group was elective major surgery (41 per cent), of whom 3.5 per cent died. Acute medical admissions were the largest emergency group (35 per cent), with a 25 per cent mortality, and emergency surgical admissions (20 per cent) had the highest death rate (28 per cent). It was found that a single 24-hour APACHE II score was not an entirely predictable guide to outcome and it was recommended that it be used with caution. There were 237 deaths (16 per cent) within the unit and a further 294 deaths (19 per cent) after discharge on the ward. This meant that 63 per cent of all patients treated were discharged from hospital alive. The high mortality occurring after discharge from the unit suggested that in many cases intensive care either did not alter the outcome or was the result, in some cases, of a clinical decision not to seek readmission to the unit when further problems arose. These cold figures marked the true impact of the success of intensive care. A few cases will illustrate this point.

A woman of 25 was pregnant with twins, but at about four months it was noted that one twin had died. Usually in cases where a single twin dies it can be resorbed and the second twin can go on to a normal birth. Unfortunately, in this case blood poisoning developed and the second twin died. Adult respiratory distress syndrome (ARDS), a state of respiratory failure, occurs as a secondary consequence of septicaemia or of other major metabolic injury such as a burn. ARDS is particularly severe in pregnancy; in this case it was so bad that at one time the patient required treatment with 100 per cent oxygen in order to obtain any gas exchange at all.

The situation appeared desperate, so we looked for other ways to treat her respiratory failure. Unfortunately, unlike the kidney, which can be replaced by the dialysis machine, at present there is no adequate mechanical replacement for the lung. It was suggested that haemofiltration might remove whatever toxin was causing the lung problem and so enable survival. This view was not widely held, but the treatment was nevertheless tried for some 36 hours, without success.

The severe ARDS problem continued, in spite of energetic treatment with antibiotics and the removal of the dead foetal material by dilatation and curettage. The patient required a tracheostomy, and the situation appeared so bad that we contacted the transplant teams with a view to considering her for a heart-lung transplant as she had suffered a single organ system failure. At that time the heart/lung transplant was technically more successful than lung transplantation alone. We were told that the only patients who would be considered for such treatment were those with chronic respiratory and cardiac conditions. We persisted in treating her with very energetic drying out of her lung tissue, including the infusion of drugs affecting blood circulation in the lung, and slowly she improved.

The pathology of ARDS is a combination of swelling of the lung tissues (oedema), inflammation and infection. Of these, oedema is perhaps the easiest to control. After some 10 weeks in the intensive care unit, the patient was weaned from the ventilator. Considering that at one stage we had proposed her for a heart/lung transplant, this represents a triumph. Her lung function has continued to improve since she was discharged from hospital, and she has made a complete recovery to normal life. The decision to persist in our efforts even though at first little progress was made was clearly right.

A fit man of 35 years, a computer expert by profession, presented with what appeared to be a chest illness at the time when there was an outbreak of Legionnaire's disease. This is an epidemic of an unusual organism, often carried in the ventilation systems of large buildings. Initially, it was thought that our patient, too, had this disease, but then he developed severe kidney failure and a rash was noticed. This was diagnosed as vasculitis (inflammation of the blood vessels), and he became extremely ill. He required assisted ventilation, as it was found that his lungs were full of blood; the vasculitic process, seemingly, had occurred in the lungs as well. This disease was treated with large doses of corticosteroid hormones and a process of blood exchange called plasmaphoresis, together with drugs to support the immune system.

After a month on the ventilator and dialysis together with very large doses of these toxic drugs, the patient made a good recovery. At the height of his illness, there were times when his lungs were so full of blood that his heart stopped – it needed to be re-started on at least three occasions. However, he basically had a curable condition, although his lungs, his kidneys and at times his heart were not working. Intensive care was able to pull him through this devastating illness. He is now well, though his kidney function has not recovered totally; it is, however, adequate to allow him to lead an entirely normal life.

We have recently reviewed the patients who suffered acute kidney failure in our intensive care unit in the last year. There were 45 patients, of whom 23 survived to leave the intensive care unit; of these, 19 left the hospital. This illustrates the need to look critically at the terms 'success' and 'survival'. Of the 19 patients who left hospital, five had essentially normal kidney function, and one who probably had underlying kidney disease needed long-term dialysis. This underlines an important fact about acute renal failure: if patients survive the illness which precipitated the kidney problem, then in most cases their kidneys will recover perfectly adequately. In fact, because such kidney failures occur as a consequence of other serious problems, usually organ system failures, most patients suffering from acute renal failure (at least in the United Kingdom) are treated in intensive care units, rather than specialized dialysis units. Another factor which has contributed to the referral of such cases to the ICU has been the development and success of haemofiltration, which is a much simpler technique to apply than haemodialysis and is readily mastered by intensive care staff. There are very few cases of acute renal failure that actually require fast haemodialysis (which is usually done in specialized dialysis units) rather than the slow form of haemodialysis which can be achieved with haemo-diafiltration.

We have tried to identify some factors which may have predicted recovery in our patients with acute kidney failure. Among these was age. There is no difference in age between those who survive and those who do not. Of course, this is a small study, and there may have been other factors which contributed to this result; but it is another indication that age on its own is not a reason for excluding patients from intensive care. Benefit from intensive care is more likely to be related to the patient's previous health and physical independence than to his age.

The last patient in this group of success stories was a 29-year-old New Zealander working in the United Kingdom. He had previously been fit and well, but suddenly suffered symptoms of fever and a severe headache. A diffuse rash developed on his body within a few hours, and he became delirious. He arrived in the accident and emergency department within four hours of the start of his symptoms and the medical registrar on duty recognized his clinical picture as being due to meningococcal meningitis. This is an acute inflammation of the meninges (membranes covering the brain), with a devastatingly high mortality. This condition has occurred in small outbreaks in various parts of the world, and in the past was responsible for the deaths of many fit, healthy young men. Cases were described in which army recruits were fit and well in the morning and dead by nightfall.

The diagnosis in this case was proved by examination of the cerebrospinal fluid by a lumbar puncture, and he was started on appropriate antibiotics. However, he developed general symptoms of septicaemia, requiring drugs to support his very low blood pressure. Kidney failure required dialysis as well; but, most worryingly, he developed signs of cardiac failure. These complications were promptly recognized. Energetic treatment, including careful monitoring of his circulation and cardiac function as well as control of fluid balance, resulted in the patient's full recovery. The keys to the success in this case were the speed at which the diagnosis was made, the clinical acumen of the duty medical registrar, and the appropriateness of the intensive care support. With patients like this it is impossible to put a price on the success of intensive care. Unfortunately, not all our cases have such a happy outcome, but clearly the successes form the inspiration and a major part of the justification for the existence of intensive care units.

# 21

# Rationing Intensive Care

I mentioned earlier that opinion, both lay and medical, has suggested that patients should not be given intensive care if they have a poor prior quality of life, and further that treatment is futile unless it can restore a normal person to full wellbeing. Both these ideas are ethically dubious at the very least and should be condemned.

There is an ever-expanding capability to prolong life and an ever-tightening budget. These two factors in combination inevitably force us to think seriously about the allocation of resources.

Medicine today faces not only a challenge to clinical autonomy but also a growing move to minimize its voice and role in health-care policy and financing. The costs of health care accelerate at a rate unacceptable to legislators and indeed to the economy in general. It is becoming vital that physicians understand and take account of cost control. It would seem preferable for economic decision-making to be made by physicians rather than for non-clinicians to make clinical decisions camouflaged as efforts at cost control.

Basically, similar principles apply in allocating any scarce medical resource. The ethicists in the Appleton Consensus made a number of suggestions, recognizing that in determining priorities with scarcity of health resources a number of concepts play critical roles.* The key principles seem to be justice and fairness of access to all patients, and selection based on medical need and possibility of medical benefit.

In practice, at my hospital rationing and restriction of access to intensive care is often decided not by intensivists but by clinicians in other parts of the hospital. They may demand intensive care for a patient after coming under pressure from a distraught family; on the other hand, they may fail to refer patients who clearly need intensive care or, worse still, refer them so late that any such treatment is futile. There comes a point, for instance in the development of multiple organ system failure, when the whole balance of body function is so disturbed that it is virtually impossible to restore. We take such patients as a challenge, even though their chances may appear extremely unpromising; surprises do occasionally occur, and it is always our concern not to deny patients the chance of recovery.

There are situations where we and other intensivists feel confident about the outcome and may be encouraged to carry on for very long periods of time. These include patients with respiratory failure. One might imagine that patients who have chronic respiratory disease might prove difficult to wean from ventilators; however, we have rarely found this to be the case. Of course, results in any medical situation may be biased by how the patients are selected for a particular treatment. Often if patients are known previously to be respiratory cripples – a condition usually defined as being housebound or even room-bound because of their inability to exert themselves owing to shortness of breath – they may well not be referred to intensive care if they develop severe respiratory problems

* Stanley, J.M., 'The Appleton Consensus', *Journal of Medical Ethics* (1989), 15 (3), 129-36.

or exacerbations of their underlying disease. The greatest difficulty we have, in fact, is to be certain that our decisions are right.

It has been suggested in some quarters that medical research and development of health care aimed at extending life should not be funded, because of social problems such treatments reveal and doubts about the quality of life in the survivors. This is not a position which I support.

The issue of age comes up in another context. It is a fact that there is an increasing percentage of elderly people in the population; and it is becoming clear that no Western country has the financial resources to provide unlimited medical care to all who need it. This inevitably leads to the conclusion that rationing of treatment will become unavoidable.

## The Oregon experiment

In the United States the state of Oregon introduced a law dealing with the high cost of medical care and the allocation of resources. It listed illnesses and conditions in order of the efficacy and cost of treatment. The list determined the order of coverage under the state Medicaid insurance programme. Professor Klein discussed this in an article.* The Oregon experiment has been widely perceived as an attempt to put medical services in some sort of objective order of priority by using the best available scientific methods. It has been both hailed as a pioneering attempt to show that resource allocation can be de-politicized, and criticized as showing a naïve faith in scientism. In fact, the most discussed and controversial aspect of the Oregon experiment – its ranking of different

---

* Klein, R., 'On the Oregon Trail: Rationing Health Care', *British Medical Journal* (1991), 302, 1-2.

forms of medical intervention in order of priority – is perhaps its least interesting aspect. In any case, the method was changed and a different list of priorities will eventually emerge, eliminating some of the perceived absurdities of priority. The real importance of the events in Oregon lies in the problems that have driven the experiment and the political processes that are shaping its progress. (It should be said that the legislation also aims to increase the number of people who have at least some medical insurance cover.)

The Oregon experiment represents an attempt to deal with a specific American problem: rationing by exclusion. It seeks to change the direction of debate from *who* is covered medically to *what conditions* are covered. In the past, Oregon sought to contain health care costs by limited eligibility for Medicaid, the American programme of last resort for the poor, and denying access, even for those eligible, to certain expensive forms of treatment, notably organ transplantation. In fact, Medicaid covers only the poor in the population – about 400,000 people out of a population of almost 3 million in the state of Oregon. Discussions about allocating funds within the Medicaid system have been held in public and on TV. The problem has been exacerbated because Oregon has imposed on itself a balanced-budget rule, so it has a very limited tax base.

The proposal for ordering medical services by priority represents a response to this crisis as well as to the more general problems of American health care, and it is an attempt to devise a financially acceptable form of universal coverage. No doubt there will be other attempts at rationing health care in an attempt to obtain the best value for money. Any form of rationing implies excluding some patients and or diseases, and this is bound to cause difficult ethical problems.

## The NHS reforms

The recent introduction of the purchaser/provider principle into the British National Health Service will have at least one uncomfortable consequence: it will focus public attention even more firmly on decisions about the level and distribution of resources, both nationally and locally. In the past decisions about who should (and should not) receive the appropriate treatment were perceived, and accepted, as matters of clinical judgement that were constrained but should not be shaped by national budgetary policies.

In future, as health authorities move towards buying packages of health care through contracts, they will increasingly have to make explicit decisions about what they want (and do not want) to buy on behalf of their local populations. Political and managerial resource-rationing priorities will therefore be visible instead of being largely hidden under the cloak of professional practices. Hence the interest in the Oregon experiment, which can be seen as the first attempt to develop an explicit system of rationing health care.*

Closer attention to cost is an important part of the National Health Service reforms of the 1990s. It will inevitably raise questions about the value of expensive therapies such as intensive care, and it may lead to rationing by cost. I have heard of a hospital where individual units are reimbursing the ICU for their patients' costs. This has led to delays in referring patients which are both dangerous and expensive: dangerous because speed in treatment is often critical; expensive because if a patient arrives in a very poor state he or she may end up needing intensive care for longer, which will of course cost more.

---

* McBride, G., 'Rationing Health Care in Oregon', *British Medical Journal* (1990), 301, 355-6.

The most efficient way to use the ICU is to treat patients early before irreversible changes have occurred.

Another method of looking at how to ration health care is by assessing outcomes – that is, the effectiveness of various medical interventions and procedures. We need to study the figures not only for vegetative survival but for functional status, cognitive function, emotional health, degree of disability, and social interaction – every aspect of 'quality of life'. In a review of 4,500 hospital records of in-patients, one-sixth of those undergoing coronary angiography and upper gastrointestinal endoscopy and one-third of those undergoing carotid endarterectomy had procedures that a consensus panel considered to be inappropriate,* obviously implying that medical practice could be improved. Such results are far more likely to occur in the United States, where there has been a much greater proliferation of coronary angiography and investigations of an invasive nature. In the United Kingdom there is less freedom of access, particularly in areas such as the treatment of coronary artery disease. I suspect that a reduction in the cost of care is part of the hidden agenda of many who promote the use of treatment guidelines.

It is recognized, however, even in the United Kingdom, that the quality of life resulting from intensive care treatment should be examined. It has been suggested by the British Intensive Care Society that we need a six-month and one-year follow-up to assess the quality of life for patients surviving intensive care. Hopefully, proper application of medical audit will answer some of these problems, improving medical care on the one hand and giving data that will help in deciding priorities for allocating resources on the other.

I believe the question of rationing of health care has been one of the reasons for the British medical

---

* Epstein, A.M., 'The Outcomes Movement', *New England Journal of Medicine* (1990), 323, 266-70.

profession's reluctance to welcome the present reorganization of the National Health Service. There is a fear that
reform will precipitate further rationing of health care in
an already depleted system. The emphasis on cost has
been seen by doctors as diverting resources from patient
care to financial control and administration. Such fears
also exist in the United States, where Professor Relman
has discussed the idea of rationing as the only effective
way to control health care costs.* The combination of a
growing ageing population, rising public health expectations and the continued introduction of new and
expensive technology generates a virtually unlimited
demand for medical treatments, which inevitably exhausts
the resources we are willing and able to devote to health
care. The question in Relman's view is not whether, but
how, health care resources will be rationed. There is
growing evidence in the United States that services are
overused, that facilities are inefficiently employed, and
that overhead and administrative expenses are excessive.
Rationing will require medical and ethical justification,
besides the need for financial restriction: rationing certain
kinds of treatment, such as kidney transplants, may well
be neither fair nor necessarily cost effective. Indeed,
cost-benefit analysis cannot even be applied to all patients.
The system needs to be improved to contain the costs.

We need to have an open discussion on resource
allocation that encompasses not only the medical
community and the source of funds, but also the moral
and ethical views of others, including the general public.
We also need an approved code of practice to maximize
the benefit to society of current limited resources.

It is clear that the question of resource allocation is
going to remain very important in a costly speciality like
intensive care because of the ever-increasing sophisti-

---

* Relman, A.S., 'The Trouble with Rationing', *New England Journal of
Medicine* (1990), 323, 911-13.

cation and expense of treatment possibilities set against finite health care budgets. These problems are apparent in both the United States and the United Kingdom and no doubt in all Western countries.

In the debate on possible rationing of resources the ICU doctor must be prepared to make the case for his speciality, and to urge that any rationing done by doctors must be based on the principles of justice and accurate medical knowledge.

The changes in the NHS make the issue of the rationing of intensive care facilities very pressing. The public needs to monitor the effects of reorganization on access to care, particularly where hospitals are being closed, and to ensure that the correct balance is maintained between relative expenditure on clinical care and administration.

# 22

# Responsibilities & Relationships

Many different skills are needed in intensive care. The director of an ICU heads a multidisciplinary team, including nurses, physiotherapists, dieticians and pharmacists as well as other doctors, such as microbiologists. The medical personnel often include a variety of specialists; usually anaesthetists predominate, but physicians and nephrologists have important roles too. It is very important to build a unified team. Morale often varies with the type of patient treated and how well the patient is faring. Paradoxically, morale is often inclined to sag at times when the unit is not busy.

Patients are admitted to hospital under the care of a physician or surgeon and then transferred to the ICU if necessary. Often the question of who is in control of the patient may give rise to differences of opinion. The intensive care doctors control the day-to-day progress, but are usually not the clinicians under whose care the patient was originally admitted. These primary clinicians may have views that differ from the intensive care team. The primary clinicians are always invited to take part in the ward rounds and in the decision-making process, but this area of communication needs to be handled with sensitivity and tact.

The decision-making process often involves a great deal

of consultation, particularly with regard to very sick patients who may die. Mutual recrimination between different teams of doctors in intensive care has to be resisted. If treatment does not succeed, or things go wrong, there is a natural tendency to look for explanations or even scapegoats. It is easy for intensive care medical staff, usually non-surgeons, to criticize surgical treatment. Surgical activities provide a high percentage of the sickest patients in intensive care – that is, those who have undergone complicated surgery or whose operations have had major complications. It is always easy to be wise after the event (doctors call it 'using the retrospectoscope'), but this is something which we try to avoid, and the best way to avoid them is by good communication.

With the reforms of the NHS of the 1990s, individual units are being encouraged to control their own budgets. This is going to increase the burden of management while also offering the opportunity for management to take place at a genuine grass-roots level. The possibility of having proper financial control of the unit may be a mixed blessing. It should be possible to purchase and plan equipment on a better basis – but only on the dubious assumption that enough money will be available. It is possible that the ICU could be asked to finance itself by cross-charging other departments of the hospital who use its resources or possibly by hiring out the unit's services to other institutions. So far these suggestions remain theoretical possibilities.

There is a case for managers of intensive care and other units to have formal training in the skills of management, which at present in the United Kingdom one is expected to pick up as one goes along. Certainly many more doctors attend management crash-courses, which must be of some benefit in the long run. One could argue, too, that management skills should be added to the list of subjects medical students are recommended to study.

It is important that proper communication occurs

between all the members of the ICU team, so that everyone's contribution is properly appreciated. Roles and responsibilities between the admitting and intensive care doctors should be clearly defined. Although in many British hospitals the fabric of the buildings is in a poor state of repair, nevertheless it is possible with good management to create a dedicated and friendly working atmosphere which is to the benefit of all concerned, not least the patients.

Attention to morale is a very important part of the ICU director's job. The prolonged presence of patients who are unlikely to survive often has an adverse effect on staff morale; standards deteriorate and the quality of care for those who can benefit is diminished as a result of staff spending much time providing treatment they suspect is ultimately going to prove futile. This does not imply that treatment withdrawal should occur because the staff feel the situation is hopeless; but it does mean that ICU decisions must be clearly explained to all concerned to ensure continuing enthusiasm and care.

The problem of adequate staffing is also a responsibility for the ICU director. I write from the fortunate position of a unit blessed with outstanding junior medical staff, but this is not a position which one can take for granted. It is also important to provide junior doctors with proper training and experience. I think that doctors undergoing postgraduate training in a variety of specialities should spend time working in the ICU. British attempts to reduce the number of junior medical staff relative to the number of consultants have serious implications for intensive care. Their declared aim is to improve career prospects for those who are accepted for hospital postgraduate training. Doctors need to be available at all times for intensive care patients. There is increasing concern over hours of duty for staff involved in life and death decisions, so it is difficult to see how reducing staff numbers is compatible with maintaining a safe level of care. I think there is an undeniable case for investing more money in intensive care.

The ICU director needs to be primarily a sensitive clinician, but he needs to have a gift for interpersonal relationships and management, in addition to an ability to make the case for increased funding of the unit as well as to plan and manage the budget. It is a formidable but an occasionally achievable combination.

### Nurse/doctor relationships

The old stereotype of the nurse/doctor relationship in which the nurse was the handmaiden of the all-knowing doctor has all but disappeared. Whether the other aspect of the nurse/doctor relationship – clandestine institutional romance between the handsome, young resident and the blushing probationer nurse – has entirely disappeared, I am no longer in a position to know.

In the old days, the doctors were in charge and the nurses were subordinate. Nowadays the relationship is a coexistence of complementary and interdependent semi-autonomous professionals. These changes reflect the changes that have taken place in the role of women in society. Nowadays approximately 50 per cent of medical school entrants are women; there is also a significant and increasing number of men in the nursing profession. Both sexes have become more adept, not only at winning the bread, but also at baking some of it at home, too.* Nowadays there is an emphasis on teamwork.

Patients' expectations of health care are now those of consumers rather than of recipients of largesse. Interestingly, there is an impression – at least in the minds of many in the medical profession – that public esteem of doctors has fallen at a time when their ability to do good has

* Editorial, 'A Suitable Case for Intimacy', *Lancet* (1990), 336, 217-18.

greatly increased; on the other hand public esteem for nurses and other health-care workers has risen. It has been difficult for both professions to handle these changes of role. Some doctors and many nurses are no longer doing what they used to do, and the people involved are often ignorant of, or misconstrue, the others' role. A doctor may feel the nurse is never there – when in fact she is sitting on some national committee; the nurse, on the other hand, may feel that the doctors do not take the patients' feelings seriously, and that they concentrate on research projects at the expense of team-building.

Other factors have led to physicians losing control over their working environment; these factors include audit, demand for second opinions, and the fact that guidelines as to treatment policy are in the process of implementation. As their control over medical practice shrinks, doctors are beginning to appreciate a kind of frustration that was previously the lot of nurses: a frustration borne of providing care for patients while having little or no control over their work.

Sometimes nurses are regarded as stubborn rebels, a view that indicates a lack of appreciation of the multiple skills demanded of nurses, particularly in intensive care, ranging from monitoring minute-by-minute physiological changes to helping patients cope with the stresses, pain and fear of chronic illness and death.* Some nurses, particularly those in some of the higher ranges of nursing academe and/or hierarchy, have claimed that the humanistic aspects of health care, such as providing health-care education, preventing disease, and helping patients and families cope with chronic illness, are the domain of nurses rather than physicians. They have also accused physicians of being addicted to the use of technology, which only increases patients' and families' need for information and support.

* Stein et al, 'Doctor/Nurse', *New England Journal of Medicine* (1990), 322, 546-9.

Nurses provide intensive care on a minute-by-minute basis, and this has made intensive care physicians uniquely dependent on them. It has also given the nurses a level of power in acute care settings that they did not enjoy previously. Doctors are inclined to accuse nurses of not accepting responsibility for the increasing conflict and dissatisfaction between physicians and their patients, but clearly there are two sides to this argument. On the other hand, it is threatening to some doctors to accept nurses as equal, competent professionals.

One of the areas in which conflict arises between doctors and nurses in my ICU is over the question of admissions. A patient may arrive when the intensive care unit is entirely full. As I mentioned in an earlier chapter (page 11), the definition of a full unit may vary. In the future there are likely to be more and more occasions when we have some empty beds but the unit is declared to be full because there are not enough nurses to staff them.

We are increasingly concerned with the stress on the nursing and medical staff because of the complexity of the tasks they have to undertake, with the inherent possibilities of error and subsequent litigation should anything go wrong. Chances of error increase with overwork. We are haunted by the fear that we are not treating all our patients for long enough.

It has been suggested that interpersonal relationships affect mortality rates in intensive care units.* On one occasion, while we were running a course for intensive care in the unit, one of the student nurses complained that our unit was unsafe because we had fallen below the norm for staffing. The situation can easily arise that patients are refused admission to intensive care because of these barriers set up by nurses. On the other hand, the nurses could argue that they have a responsibility to manage the

---

* Knaus, W.A., 'Outcome in ITU', *Annals of Internal Medicine* (1986), 104, 410-18.

patients and if anything goes wrong they will be held responsible. In fact, the result of this student nurse's complaint was a very tiresome and prolonged inquiry causing great distress to the staff nurses involved. Whether in fact it did any good is doubtful; we hope, however, that our admission policy will help prevent such a thing happening in the future.

The clear need in resolving the nurse/doctor battle is for good communication on a continuous basis, and this is what we try to achieve in my own unit. In fact doctors and nurses may, or should, receive similar training in social areas such as helping families to cope with sickness and bereavement. Leadership can emerge in hierarchies allocating talented expertise to particular tasks. This, and good communication, should result in better treatment for the patient.

The roles of doctor and nurse in intensive care, although converging in many respects, retain their differences. The key to success in the unit is to integrate the disciplines into a unified team with mutual respect and understanding. There needs to be a flexibility of approach on both sides and a readiness to alter working patterns. I can see no reason why the manager or director of the unit need always be a doctor rather than a nurse. The aim must always be to achieve the best possible care for the patient, and this means utilizing all the available talents in the ICU to their fullest potential.

# 23

## Legal Problems

A significant percentage of the critically ill patients admitted to intensive care will die. When one of these patients dies, however hopeless the medical situation may have been there is always a tendency for relatives to wonder if something went wrong with the care of their loved one – a failure to give the correct treatment, for instance, or make the correct diagnosis. Withdrawal of treatment in intensive care is another area where the possibility of legal action always exists. There are many situations when, because of the emergency and the critical nature of problems arising in intensive care, it would be impractical to attempt to obtain consent and hence to delay or deny life-saving treatment. The question of consent is usually more a theoretical than a real problem.

The legal issues in intensive care are much less clearly defined in the United Kingdom than in the United States. In the United States many problems in medicine and indeed in other fields can be resolved in the courts, having evolved either out of classical common law concepts or as questions of constitutional rights of the individual. British medicine is more paternalistic: a doctor is required to tell a patient only what any reasonable doctor would disclose; in other words he does not have to tell the patients all the details of his case. In America the courts have held that patients should be informed consumers, so doctors must disclose at least all that a 'reasonable patient' would want to know.

In the United States it is a well established principle that patients have the right to refuse treatment and that surrogates can refuse for them. In the Cruzan case (pages 54-6), the Supreme Court articulated the existence of this right to refuse life-sustaining treatment, including the feeding which was included as a medical treatment. In the United States the concept and use of the living will has developed (page 89), enabling people to give detailed directions, binding in law, on how they want to be treated if and when they become incapacitated. Thse directives are made when the person is of a sound mind.

In the United States federal legislation requires hospitals and nursing homes to tell a patient of his state's laws relating to consenting or refusing life-support treatment under the Patient Self-Determination Act (it must be remembered that the laws vary from state to state within the Union). Some states allow patients to refuse treatment that would prolong their lives if they become incapacitated. Patients must receive written information regarding their rights at the time of admission and a note must be made in the patient's record as to whether the patient has rejected life support. A number of the states allow health-care proxies.

Personally, I am concerned about both the living will, and, even more, about the legislation where patients are asked to make statements about their treatment preferences. In concept these laws are designed as instruments of consumer information and protection. In practice they may cause the patient additional stress and anxiety.

The living will may in fact discourage organizations and hospitals from treating people with curable conditions, and it may be very difficult to prove whether a patient was actually of sound mind when he signed such a will. The law assumes that a patient will not change his views when the need actually arises. The idea of presenting patients coming into hospital with documents reminding them that they have rights not to be treated seems a little absurd. I would guess that most patients would not want such measures to be applied to them, and I would also guess that many of the patients who are admitted to hospital are in no state to make such decisions because of distress, confusion or pain. All too many of them, particularly in inner city areas, have no obvious surrogate who could reliably do this for them. There are other drawbacks to the legalistic framework of medical treatment in the United States; in particular medical decisions may be affected or determined by unspoken pressure to avoid lawsuits.

It is ironic that, although patients' rights are legally protected in the United States, a significant proportion of patients unfortunately fall through the health care network because they have inadequate or no health insurance, a situation which does not occur if there is a well-funded state health service. Sadly, this does not entirely apply in the United Kingdom either at present.

Litigation for negligence in the United Kingdom has greatly increased in recent years. In addition the Crown Prosecuting Service brings criminal charges against people whose professional mistakes cost lives. An act of negligence which results in a patient's death can now expose a doctor to a civil action for negligence. The doctor could also face a General Medical Council disciplinary hearing and National Health Service Complaints Procedures. The combination of these proceedings would in most cases end the doctor's professional career. It seems excessive to add the extra burden of a trial for manslaughter.

There have been trials for manslaughter of doctors who gave an anti-cancer drug by the wrong route – into the cerobrospinal fluid instead of the vein. Personally I felt the consultant concerned, rather than the hapless juniors, should have been accused. In 1990, a senior house officer (junior resident) was cleared of murdering a terminally ill cancer patient with a drug injection which his lawyer said was to kill the pain and not the patient. One can readily envisage such actions occurring in relation to real or perceived errors in intensive care.

I believe that the situation in the United Kingdom concerning the legal framework in intensive care is moving in the same direction as in the United States. In Britain various committees and working parties make recommendations which set the standard for medical practice. The Institute of Medical Ethics Working Party on the Ethics of Prolonging Life and Assisting Death recommended that doctors may sometimes be ethically justified in assisting the death of a patient in continued pain or distress caused by an incurable illness and who has expressed a clear and consistent wish for this previously.* In fact the legal position in the United Kingdom is unclear, mainly because there has been much less discussion of the issues than in the United States. Similarly unclear is the legal position regarding withdrawing treatment in patients in whom intensive care is not achieving any progress.

In a further report this working party urged professional bodies to recognize publicly that withdrawal of artificial nutrition and hydration may be an appropriate way to manage vegetative patients. The availability of such declarations by professional bodies would enable individual doctors to raise such a possibility sensitively with relatives and would promote discussion of this difficult subject between professional carers and the public. Whether such statements by advisory committees will subsequently be codified into law is a different matter, but they do at least provide backing for the doctors who have

---

* Institute of Medical Ethics Working Party, 'Withdrawal of Life Support', *Lancet* (1990), 336, 610-13.

to make these difficult decisions. The ethics and conditions of treatment withdrawal merit public debate.

This problem of the legality as well as the ethics of withdrawing treatment may arise not only in the ICU but also in patients who have been in the intensive care unit but have recovered only to a persistent vegetative state rather than to true wellbeing. These decisions are taken in the wards by the doctors in charge after discussion and with the consent of the family. I have tried to avoid being a party to them, but this may be a cowardly approach.

That there clearly are moves to define the legal position regarding withholding treatment in Britain is shown by the fact that Lord Donaldson, Master of the Rolls, gave a judgement (see page 119) in the Court of Appeal in October 1990, on whether a severely handicapped 5-month-old baby should be allowed to die.

The advance of medical technology has led to the raising of legal issues in relation to medical treatment in many countries. In France Dr Schwartzenberg, a well-known oncologist, was found in breach of an article of the doctor's code of professional ethics according to which a physician must abstain from any act likely to reflect upon the honour of the profession. Some three years previously he had given an interview in which he had stated that a patient had the right to a dignified death. He also had stated that he had helped patients in great pain and in a desperate condition to die. He was suspended by the Conseil d'Etat in France.

In Israel in 1990, doctors caring for a patient with amyotrophic lateral sclerosis, which is a currently incurable condition of progressive deterioration of function of all the muscles and nerves, associated with progressive weakness and wasting, wanted court assistance in order to protect themselves from possible charges of manslaughter which might arise if they granted a patient's request for limitation of treatment. The court accepted the patient's videotaped request not to be attached to a life-support machine when his condition deteriorated to such a state that this would appear to be needed. This implied that the doctors could not be charged with manslaughter or negligence for not initiating life support in line with the patient's recorded wishes.

There is considerable anxiety about the possibility of lawsuits for negligence or worse arising in intensive care. There are fears that one patient's compensation may prevent another patient's treatment unless the public is prepared to increase health-care expenditure or to limit claims. Because of the limitations on resources it is conceivable that large settlements for medical accidents in intensive care may result in certain attempts at life-saving being considered too hazardous to attempt because of the danger of litigation. I do not think this has yet happened in Britain but it is a possibility.

The report of the King's Fund has suggested standardizing treatment and providing protocols for all treatments in intensive care. One of the benefits of this would be to set standards against which practice could be measured. I hope we will be able to maintain the traditional level of mutual trust between doctors, patients and the family that has been a feature of British medical practice.

We try to forestall medico-legal problems in my unit by detailed discussion of progress with the patient or his nearest and dearest, particularly when issues such as withholding further treatment arise. Frequently a case conference is arranged where all the physicians and surgeons concerned with the patient as well as the nurses meet with the patient's family. We hope that by such practice the chances of our facing a legal challenge of our actions are diminished, and it gives an opportunity for all concerned to discuss their views and resolve any emotional and ethical doubts. Failure of adequate communication with the relatives is often the prime cause of legal action by the bereaved.

# Conclusion

The purpose of this book has been to try to inform the public of the ethical dilemmas faced in intensive care. There has been a very rapid expansion in the ability of medicine to treat and even cure what was considered hopeless only a few short years ago. This has increased public demand for medical treatment and has consequently led to a steady increase in costs of health care. When is it ethically permissible to withhold, let alone withdraw, medical treatment? Should we persist in trying novel experimental treatments in people who are obviously dying?

The doctor in intensive care must always bear in mind the cardinal principles of medical ethics, namely, that he or she is there to benefit the patient not to harm him. He has to respect the patient's autonomy and his actions must be just. As far as benefit is concerned, the question of when it is of benefit to the patient to withdraw and/or withhold treatment remains a constant source of ethical anxiety. The age of medical paternalism has all but passed and the need to respect the patient's autonomy is established. It is ethically very difficult to accept this autonomy when, if exercised, it will actually lead to harm, at least in the majority view of the body of medical opinion. In fact the status of patient autonomy is being refined all the time by legal cases on issues such as forced feeding of people with anorexia nervosa, or giving blood transfusions to Jehovah's Witnesses. The question of

197

fairness in intensive care comes up in terms of access of patients to this specialized treatment. It is often tempting to exclude certain diagnostic categories on a blanket basis and this is ethically repugnant.

The interface between economics and ethics is becoming increasingly important. Is it ethical for patients' lives not to be saved because there isn't enough money? Or is it wrong to save just a few lives when the same money could give a lesser degree of benefit to many people? Because of escalating costs, many changes are being made in the delivery of healthcare; changes which I suspect have little or nothing to do with benefit and everything to do with saving money. It is vital that the general public monitors these changes.

There is undoubtedly a need for intensive care to be as economical as possible. To this end it may be necessary to amalgamate intensive care units into larger entities as this will cut down overheads and running costs, but for this to be ethically permissible would entail an efficient and safe means of transportation to these units, which may be separated by long distances. It is important that the public makes its views known. Adequate facilities and resources for intensive care need to be demanded by the public, who should also demand proper accountability. If doctors ask for increased resources they are frequently accused of shroud-waving, scare-mongering or worse. The medical profession must explain the place and value of intensive care so the public will support our efforts. There is a need also for the public to become aware of the ethical problems and, indeed, to express their views. This is not always the case today and it is only with the support and help of the public that intensive care can give the service which the public deserves. Britain is already underprovided in terms of ICU facilities as compared with other European countries. The public must help the medical profession with political support to maintain health services including intensive care by adequate funding. It is important that the public is able to discuss and indeed express views about these ethical dilemmas so that it is the general public rather than the doctor who controls life in line with the patient's principles and beliefs.

# Index